THE
DIABETIC'S
BOOK

Also by June Biermann and Barbara Toohey:

The Woman's Holistic Headache Relief Book
The Diabetic's Sports and Exercise Book
The Peripatetic Diabetic
The Diabetic Woman (with Lois Jovanovic, M.D.)
The Diabetic's Total Health Book

THE DIABETIC'S BOOK

All Your Questions Answered

JUNE BIERMANN

and

BARBARA TOOHEY

JEREMY P. TARCHER, INC.
Los Angeles

Library of Congress Cataloging in Publication Data

Biermann, June.
   The diabetic's book : all your questions answered / June Biermann
and Barbara Toohey.
     p.   cm.
   Includes bibliographical references.
   1. Diabetes—Miscellanea. I. Toohey, Barbara. II. Title.
RC660.B459 1990
616.4'62—dc20   89-20366
   ISBN 0-87477-552-3 (pbk.)   CIP

Jeremy P. Tarcher, Inc.
5858 Wilshire Blvd., Suite 200
Los Angeles, CA 90036

Distributed by St. Martin's Press, New York

Design by Tanya Maiboroda

Manufactured in the United States of America
10 9 8 7 6 5 4

To Jackie Tippen,
who over the last thirty years
has given us the two greatest gifts:
love and work.

Contents

All things are difficult
before they are easy.

—THOMAS FULLER, 1608–1661
Gnomologia No. 560

Foreword

. . . .

An old Talmudic saying goes "All beginnings are difficult." This couldn't be more true for persons with diabetes. To begin life over as a diabetic person is not only difficult but slightly short of impossible. Receiving the diagnosis of diabetes has nearly the same jolt as seeing your whole life—your inner house—collapse after an earthquake or hurricane.

The Diabetic's Book: All Your Questions Answered can be your guide to that new beginning. June and Barbara will lead you through the rebuilding and healing process with sound advice, knowledge, and wisdom gained over many years. They take the guilt out of "getting" the disease. It is hard to move forward when fear, anxiety, and anger are all pushing you back. Diabetes self-care necessitates information, skill, and concentration. This book provides it all.

Let me tell you why I feel so strongly about this tome.

First, it truly answers all your questions, as the title suggests. I know of few other books on diabetes that contain the wealth of information you will find here. The advice and facts are not only up-to-date but are substantiated by an extensive literature review and the secondary opinions of many leading experts in the field of diabetes self-care. June and Barbara also give you their own firsthand experiences and those of many other real people who live with diabetes day in and day out.

Second, this book teaches you the basic language of diabetes in a clear and straightforward manner. Each and every time a medical term is used, it is explained and defined. This is no small feat. One of the worst complications of diabetes is actually the misunderstandings that frequently occur between diabetic patients and their health-care team. Thus, your new language skill will mean that the important communication between you and your doctor and dietician can begin.

Third, this work speaks to every diabetic, regardless of whether you are Type I or Type II (you will learn the difference in the first section), young or old, in control or out of control. I am particularly pleased with the coverage June and Barbara have provided for the person with Type II diabetes who is so often forgotten in other books on diabetes. In the past, Type II diabetes was thought to be a mild disorder that did not demand attention to blood glucose control. Today, we now know that Type II diabetes needs the full respect that Type I diabetes always had. Those of you with Type II diabetes need to keep your blood glucose levels as near to normal as possible to avoid the complications of diabetes. To achieve this goal, the Type II diabetic must adhere to diet, medication, exercise, and blood-sugar monitoring. This change in the philosophy of Type II diabetes treatment and self-care is clearly explained and beautifully chronicled by June and Barbara.

Fourth, there is a level of detail in this book that is unmatched in other beginner diabetes manuals. In every section, Barbara and June provide tiny gems of information that one generally does not find elsewhere. From diet tips to exercise hints to insulin injection equipment to advice for parents and families, you will find dozens of ideas that can truly make life easier for all involved.

From their suggestions, I learned to watch business trends for the latest breakthrough developments in diabetes control and treatment. Barbara and June are so right about this. After all, it only makes sense that we will learn about new discoveries and inventions in the pages of the *Wall Street Journal* and other business magazines before new diabetes products hit the market.

By staying abreast of the business news, every diabetic person can follow the research done at dozens of companies and thereby feel a bit more hopeful that a cure is on the way.

Lastly, and perhaps most important, this book will motivate you to make the necessary changes in your life to live well with diabetes. As you read these pages, I am sure you will feel, as I did, that you are in good hands and that you have been truly understood. Through their own experiences with diabetes, Barbara and June know the ins and outs of depression, frustration, and fear. They write sensitively about what every diabetic person and concerned family member goes through, and they teach you how to have a sense of humor about it. It is easier to laugh when you know you are not alone, and diabetes is so much more tolerable to live with when you can laugh about dietary restrictions, injections, blood tests, mood swings, and annoying itches. June and Barbara will almost make you feel sorry for persons who do not have diabetes!

You will also find that this book can motivate your family and friends to a new beginning as well. The section addressed to them is worth the price of the book alone. Not only will they start to understand your diabetes, but they will gain a new sense of themselves and the role they can play in helping you to live a full and satisfied life rather than, as often happens, making "your" problem "their" problem.

When you have finished reading these pages, I am sure you will agree with my sentiments about this wonderful book. Thank you, June and Barbara. I enjoyed, I learned, I identified with all you have to offer here. Bravo for your new edition of *The Diabetic's Book*. All my questions *were* answered.

Lois Jovanovic-Peterson, M.D.
Senior Scientist, Sansum Medical Research Foundation,
Santa Barbara, California
Clinical Professor of Medicine,
University of Southern California,
Los Angeles

Introduction

. . . .

Although this book is intended for anyone involved with diabetes—whether a newly diagnosed or experienced diabetic, a family member or friend, or a diabetes health professional—it is aimed primarily at beginners.

Why beginners? For two reasons. The first was born one day when the June half of our writing team was emerging from her dentist's office. The door to a neighboring internist's office opened and a man came out. He was clutching a copy of the American Diabetes Association's approved diet, *Exchange Lists for Meal Planning*.

The man had obviously just been given *the news*, because in ninety-six-point headlines his face was printed with confusion, fear, and despair. June could read these emotions easily because they were the same ones she'd seen in the mirror on her own D (for *diagnosis*) day. While writing this book, we've kept this man's face before us. Our goal has been to change his expression—and that of all newly diagnosed diabetics—to one of understanding, courage, and hope.

The second reason for aiming this book at beginners is based on the Zen theory of the expert's mind versus the beginner's mind. Since the expert's mind thinks it knows everything, it is closed to new ideas. It knows what *can't* be done. It thinks in terms of limitations. The beginner's mind, on the other hand, is still open. To the beginner all things are possible. Not even the sky is the limit.

1

We hope that this book will help all of you—no matter how many years you've had diabetes or have worked in the field of diabetes—to become beginners again.

The Diabeticization of America

In the nine years since the original publication of *The Diabetic's Book*, America has been what we might call "diabeticized." The estimated number of diagnosed diabetics has risen from under 10 million to over 12 million, and there could be an equal number out there undiagnosed. As the population ages and longevity increases, the incidence of diabetes correspondingly goes up. Today, almost 18 percent of the population between the ages of sixty-five and seventy-four has diabetes, and few would be surprised to see this number double in the next twenty-five years.

As a result of this new recognition of diabetes as a burgeoning health problem, new products and therapies have been developed to make diabetes care easier and more effective. Now instead of two blood-sugar meters there are ten; instead of one automatic injector for insulin there are five. Insulin infusion pumps have shrunk to the size of a pack of cards, and formerly complex jet injectors are now simple enough for children to operate.

But the diabeticization of America is having an impact everywhere. Because of dramatic increases in medical costs for all Americans, there is a newfound interest across the entire country in health, and self-care and preventive maintenance, always the cornerstones of a successful diabetes regimen, have become the way of life for everyone.

For example, we might say that the American diet has been diabeticized. The diabetic diet, formerly considered unusual and difficult to impose on the rest of the family, is now recognized as the ideal diet for everyone and is endorsed by the American Heart Association, the American Cancer Society, the surgeon general, and many reputable weight-loss programs. New sugar-free, low-fat, high-fiber, low-sodium foods have appeared on the market to make it not only convenient to follow that diet but a pleasure as well.

With the increased research and understanding of diabetes in the eighties, a new optimism, a *realistic* optimism about the disease reigns. In February 1989, the *Journal of the American Medical Association* finally acknowledged something that well-informed diabetes health professionals and well-controlled diabetics have known and acted on for years: *keeping blood sugar normal will prevent the dreaded complications of diabetes.* And a cure, while perhaps not just down the block, is at least visible on the horizon.

Yes, things are very much better now than they were back in 1965, when June was diagnosed diabetic. Although it was not the worst of times to become diabetic, it was not the best of times, either. Practical help for those with this health problem was scarce. The now active and growing American Association of Diabetes Educators (six thousand members) didn't even exist. The available books were ponderous and discouraging. Those greatest tools for keeping your blood sugar under control—home blood-sugar-testing meters—hadn't been invented. Diabetics were condemned to use notoriously inaccurate and distressingly unaesthetic urine tests. They often had only monthly or quarterly or even, in some cases, annual blood-sugar tests in the doctor's office.

Because of this lack of help, information, and effective technology, we started devoting a considerable portion of our time to finding strategies for coping with diabetes. Using June as a guinea pig, we constantly checked out new angles of attack on the problems of living with diabetes. In conversations after our talks at diabetes associations, and in correspondence with hundreds of other diabetics and health professionals, we continued to learn more. We shared our newfound, ever-expanding (and changing) store of information in our previous books on diabetes: *The Peripatetic Diabetic* in 1969 (revised in 1984), *The Diabetes Question and Answer Book* in 1974, *The Diabetic's Sports and Exercise Book* in 1977, *The Diabetic's Total Health Book* in 1980 (revised in 1988), the first edition of *The Diabetic's Book: All Your Questions Answered* in 1981, and *The Diabetic Woman* in 1987.

Because it is our most basic and accessible book on diabetes and because it has been used as a teaching text in many diabetes education programs, *The Diabetic's Book* has been read by more people than any of our other books on the subject: over sixty thousand copies are out there somewhere in diabetesland. Of course, it made us happy to be able to reach and, we hope, *teach* so many of those involved with diabetes.

But in the last couple of years we started cringing at the thought of how out-of-date the book had become. There has never been a period in the history of diabetes in which so many new discoveries—all to the good—have been made and so much new information has become available on how people with diabetes can make their lives easier, happier, healthier, and *longer*. We needed to capture all that and put it into a revised edition.

In addition, over the last nine years, we've been in contact with thousands of diabetics and their families and with many doctors, nurses, dietitians, psychologists, social workers, and exercise therapists specializing in diabetes, particularly because of our work at the SugarFree Centers, where we supply diabetics with the latest in self-therapy equipment, products, and learning materials. All of these people have generously shared with us their insights and innovations.

Now at last we can bring all this newfound knowledge and inspiration to you. Even as we write this revision, though, we experience bittersweet feelings—bitter because we know that new developments in diabetes are constantly emerging, new breakthroughs are announced almost daily, and it won't be long before we start cringing again at the out-of-date aspects of the book. The sweet part is that every development and every breakthrough will be a step toward better understanding and an eventual cure of the disease. To keep you informed of these beneficial changes as we learn them, we invite you to call or write for a copy of the SugarFree Centers' newsletter, *Health-O-Gram* (in California, 1-800-336-1222; in the rest of the U.S., 1-800-972-2323; Box 114,

Van Nuys, California 91408). Health professionals should also request the *Professional Info-Gram*.

In revising this book we have kept in mind that it is for the reader who has recently been diagnosed and who undoubtedly has many concerns and questions. We also have thought about the use of this text in educational programs. Therefore, in writing style and organization, we remain guided by the needs of both audiences. We've kept our original goals of readability and accuracy plus a touch of fun and a feel for the human condition. We hope this new edition will continue to be a flexible learning tool equally useful with individuals and groups and that diabetes teaching teams will find it even more compatible with their own creative classroom techniques.

We've made one important change in organization. In the first edition we had three sections: questions and answers for everyone, questions and answers for Type I (insulin-dependent) diabetics, and questions and answers for family members and friends. In this edition, we've added a section of questions and answers for that great and often neglected—alas, even by us— group, the Type II's (non-insulin-dependent). We recognize here that this group, which comprises the majority of diabetics, has almost a different disease from the Type I's, with unique problems resulting in unique questions with unique answers.

All in all, we feel that if you had to become diabetic, this is the best time in the history of the world for it to happen. Never before has it been so possible to keep your blood sugar normal, to avoid (or reverse or minimize) the feared complications of diabetes, and to enjoy life as it was meant to be enjoyed. With this book we want you to learn how to live better with diabetes and *through* diabetes.

June Biermann
Barbara Toohey
Van Nuys, California
February 1990

Something for Everyone

The old saying "You can't see the forest for the trees" is, like many such sayings, very true. Sometimes you're so close to the individual aspects of a problem, you can't see the whole picture. And not seeing the whole picture may prevent you from gaining the perspective necessary to attain overall control of the situation.

Therefore, before we launch into the specifics of how to take care of yourself as an insulin-taking or non-insulin-taking diabetic, or how to master the emotional aspects of the disease and manage your daily life, or how to offer the best support possible for your diabetic family member or friend, we'll take a look at the big picture of diabetes. This is what everyone needs to know. You'll find that once you see the forest of diabetes, you'll find it easier to get out of the woods.

DIABETES AND CONTROL

What is diabetes?

Diabetes is a physical problem that causes you to have too much sugar in your blood. The medical name for it is *diabetes mellitus*.

7

The first word, *diabetes*, is from Greek and means "to run through a siphon." The second word, *mellitus*, is from Latin, and means "honey." The two words together are usually translated "sweet water siphon." (In case you don't speak Greek and Latin, *diabetes mellitus* is pronounced *dye-uh-**beet**-ease **mell**-uh-tus*.) The doctors in ancient times called it that because they noticed that diabetics urinated a great deal and that their urine tasted sweet. Yes, *tasted* sweet. In those days the only way a doctor could test urine was by tasting it. (And doctors today won't even make house calls!)

Diabetes can be broken down into Type I (insulin-dependent) and Type II (non-insulin-dependent). Type I is the newer term for what used to be called juvenile-onset diabetes, because it occurs most frequently in people under twenty years old. In actuality, Type I diabetes affects people over twenty also. For instance, June got diabetes as an adult in her forties, but she has to take insulin. Sometimes people like her are referred to as Type I½'s. Her pancreas still produces some insulin but not enough, while in true Type I's the pancreas produces no insulin.

Type II is the current term for what used to be called adult-onset diabetes. We now know that Type II diabetes is not limited to people over forty, as used to be thought, but that it occurs in teenagers and even in some children. According to Stanley Mirsky, M.D., author of *Controlling Diabetes the Easy Way*, about 5 percent of Type II's are under twenty years of age.

Type I and Type II diabetes have such a number of differences that some experts theorize that they are actually two different diseases. But with both types there is the problem of too much sugar in the blood.

There is also a kind of diabetes that has nothing to do with blood sugar. It's called *diabetes insipidus*, and it is a problem of the hypothalamus rather than the pancreas. The hypothalamus produces an antidiuretic hormone that limits the formation of urine in the kidneys. When something (tumor, infection, or injury) damages the hypothalamus, interfering with the production of the hormone, excessive urination (along with excessive water drinking) is the result.

Diabetes insipidus can be hereditary and, like diabetes mellitus, can be controlled by the use of a hormone. Strangely enough, this hormone is sometimes taken in the form of a nasal spray. (Too bad insulin can't be snorted in this way!)

Diabetes insipidus is also called "water diabetes" to differentiate it from "sugar diabetes."

Why is there too much sugar in the blood?

The cells of the body run on a fuel called *glucose*. This is the sugar that the body manufactures from the food we eat. Glucose is carried to the cells in the bloodstream, but if you have diabetes it cannot be absorbed because the cells are locked up tighter than a Manhattan apartment. Glucose can't get into a cell without a key. That key is *insulin*. Insulin is a hormone that comes from a gland called the pancreas. The particular cells of the pancreas that produce insulin are the beta cells.

In Type I diabetes the beta cells have been totally destroyed and make no insulin, or have been partially destroyed and don't make enough insulin (Type I½). That is to say, all or some of the insulin keys are missing so they can't let the sugar into the cells. Such people will need to inject insulin, which we will explain later.

In Type II diabetes, the beta cells are still there perking along, manufacturing plenty of insulin keys, but either the cells in the bloodstream don't have enough locks (called insulin receptors) for the insulin key to fit in, or something is keeping the locks from working. (This is called insulin resistance or insulin insensitivity.) These people will need to modify their diet, lose weight, and make other changes to control their diabetes. We will also explain this treatment shortly.

In both cases, the result is that sugar is left in the bloodstream, causing high blood sugar.

There is a convenient test doctors use to determine whether

a diabetic still makes any insulin and roughly how much. It is called a C-peptide test and is a blood test ordinarily taken after overnight fasting and before breakfast. The more insulin your body makes, the higher your C-peptide level. The level of blood-serum C-peptide is usually zero in Type I diabetics. In Type II's it can be within or above the normal range.

What's wrong with having high blood sugar?

High blood sugar is an indication that your body is getting little or no fuel. In desperation it begins to convert its own fat and muscle into fuel. This is like chopping down the walls of your house to get wood to burn in your fireplace. If you keep that up, soon you have no house left.

But that's not even the worst of it. When the body burns itself for fuel, excess *ketones* (substances that are formed during the digestion of fat) are given off. These excess ketones can poison the body. This poisoning—called *ketoacidosis*—can lead to death. You may remember the television program about the California boy Wesley Parker, whose father threw away his insulin because a faith healer had "cured" the boy's disease. Within three days Wesley was dead from ketoacidosis.

There is also something else wrong with having high blood sugar. Let's say you have *some* insulin that's working—either insulin you've injected or insulin you've produced in your own pancreas—but you don't have enough. Or say you have plenty of insulin but it's not able to get the sugar into the cells. Then, while you won't use up your own body as fuel and you won't be poisoning yourself with ketones, you still have too much sugar flowing through your bloodstream. That's not good, because this situation brings about long-range diabetes complications like blindness, kidney failure, and gangrene of the feet.

What caused me to get diabetes?

Researchers have been puzzling over the answer to this question for decades. They have more leads now than ever before but still not many definite answers. We'll summarize points of what is known, and you'll have to try to apply them to yourself.

First, diabetes runs in families; so whether you got it as a child or later in life, you still had to have some genes that predisposed you to it. Second, some physical or emotional stresses combined with your hereditary tendency and possibly your environment pushed you over the brink into diabetes.

If you got Type I diabetes as a child (the commonest age to be diagnosed is around twelve), recent studies show that a virus related to the mumps virus might have begun damaging your pancreatic cells that produce insulin. This triggered an immune response so that your body's own immune system continued the destruction until after several years your insulin-producing capability was totally gone and you had diabetes. Scientists also suspect a strong environmental factor in childhood diabetes, since the highest incidence is in areas where the climate is the coldest and more cases are diagnosed in the winter than in the summer.

For those diagnosed in midlife or later, the Type II's, the number-one diabetes-triggering stress is excess weight. Some 80 to 85 percent of those diagnosed are overweight. Another influence is aging and a general slowing of body functions. In fact, more cases of diabetes are diagnosed after the age of sixty than at any other time of life.

Overproduction of certain hormones—growth hormone from the pituitary, thyroid hormone, epinephrine, cortisone, and glucagon—makes the body's insulin less effective and can also bring on diabetes.

Pregnancy, which makes additional demands on the body, can cause diabetes to develop. In fact, some women show diabetes symptoms during pregnancy but their symptoms disappear after the baby is delivered. (This is called gestational diabetes.) Mary Tyler Moore wasn't that lucky. Her diabetes was diagnosed shortly after a miscarriage, and from then on she has been insulin-dependent.

Surgery or a major illness can activate diabetes. June became diabetic not long after a hysterectomy.

And finally, emotional stress has been implicated. This can be either long-term, grinding stress such as chronic unhappiness with a job or a family situation, or it can be a sudden extreme emotional shock. One woman we know became diabetic almost immediately after her husband was killed in an automobile accident.

Many people have the mistaken idea that they can get diabetes from eating too many sweets. (As we said, diabetes is sometimes called "sugar diabetes," which adds to the confusion.) Diabetes can't be caused by eating too much sugar, except when your diabetes was triggered by overweight and you became overweight from eating too many sweets. But even in that case, it wasn't specifically the sugar that was to blame. Diabetes could have developed if you ate too much of anything and gained weight.

Why didn't I have any symptoms of diabetes when my case was diagnosed?

You were one of the thousands of hidden diabetics—people who have diabetes and don't realize it. You're one of the smart (or lucky) ones. You caught diabetes early, before it had done any real damage.

If you neglect your diabetes in the future, you may begin to experience the classic symptoms of the acute stages of diabetes: excessive urination and thirst, increased appetite, rapid loss of weight, irritability, weakness, fatigue, nausea, and vomiting. These indicate ketoacidosis, which if untreated will lead to coma and ultimately death. These are the symptoms that usually strike children and adolescents suddenly.

Most people who get Type II diabetes after the age of twenty have a different set of symptoms, though they may also have any of the above. Generally, the warning signals are drowsiness, itching, blurred vision, tingling and numbness in the feet, fatigue, skin infections, and slow healing. Type II diabetics often have two additional clues that diabetes may be in the offing: they are overweight, and they have a family history of diabetes.

Can diabetes be cured?

Not yet. So that means you have diabetes for the rest of your life unless there is a breakthrough. We can report, however, that things are looking up. The good news for Type II's is that two pathologists in Minnesota working with doctors in Sweden have reported the discovery of a polypeptide (a chain of amino acids linked together) that inhibits the ability of cells to take in sugar and physically destroys the insulin-making islet cells. This polypeptide could be the prime agent responsible for Type II diabetes or a contributor to its development. And just in case these researchers are not onto something big, we have an encouraging prediction from Dr. Rachmiel Levine, emeritus physician at the City of Hope Hospital in California. He believes the oral drugs will eventually do the total job of control for most Type II's.

Meanwhile, scientists are working on a number of promising possibilities for the cure and/or better control of Type I diabetes.

Beta cell transplants. Here is where the most hope lies at the moment. Human or pork (fetal or synthetic) beta cell islets that are protected against antibody invasion by a special membrane have been developed at the University of California Medical Center at San Francisco. These are transplanted into your body to take over for your destroyed beta cells. According to Dr. Peter H. Forsham, emeritus professor there, the process has been patented and could be available as early as 1992. It could be the ultimate solution, at least for Type I diabetes.

Pancreas transplants. More than fifteen hundred pancreas transplants have been performed throughout the world, with a success rate of between 40 and 80 percent. So far, the transplants have been performed mainly on diabetics who have a kidney transplant and are already taking immunosuppressive drugs to keep the kidney from being rejected, since the same drugs will keep the pancreas from being rejected.

We met one young South Carolinan, forty-four-year-old Mary Ellen Baran, who had a transplant in 1972, after twenty-three years as a diabetic. She was cured of diabetes. We had breakfast with Mary Ellen in Atlanta once and watched in amazement as she relished her pancakes and syrup. She confessed that "within three months of leaving the hospital, I had tested every dessert known to man and gained fifteen pounds." She now has a grip on her new freedom, and her weight is back to normal. "My meal plans are *exactly* as they were before the operation," she told us. And believe it or not, she says she eats less refined sugar now than she did as a diabetic.

A mechanical pancreas. A small implantable artificial "beta cell" is on the drawing boards. The device has an insulin reservoir and a pump, a power supply, a glucose sensor, and a computer. Problems with the sensor are holding back the appearance of this system, but as soon as these are overcome this could become available.

Keep watching the papers. You'll be seeing a lot of headlines like "Diabetes Cure in Sight." Unfortunately, when you read on, you'll probably discover that the "fantastic" breakthrough has been with three mice in New Jersey.

In time, however, we're confident that a real cure will come. What you have to do in the meantime is keep your spirits up, keep your diabetes under control, and keep yourself in the best possible shape so that you'll be able to, as Mary Ellen puts it, "hop onto your own star when it comes your way."

Will diabetes shorten my life?

In the past the statistics about the shortened life expectancy of diabetics have been, to say the least, depressing. The old estimate of life expectancy for diabetics was that, *all things being equal*, diabetes shortens a person's life by one-third. But that estimate is now questionable because of the advent of blood-sugar testing and the immense increase in the number of people who are in good control. But for the sake of argument, let's accept it. What, then, does "all things being equal" mean?

Our interpretation is that if you do *not* have diabetes and yet you live the way diabetics do—you eat a perfectly balanced diet low in fats and sugar; you drink little or no alcohol; you do not smoke; you keep your weight slightly below normal; you get regular daily exercise and regular nightly sleep—you will live one-third longer than a diabetic doing the same thing.

But let's face it. Without the incentive of a chronic health problem to make them follow such an optimum lifestyle, ninety-nine people out of one hundred won't do it. No, better make that 999,999 out of 1 million.

Now, let's say all things *aren't* equal. You don't have diabetes. You are overeating—and eating all the wrong things—over-drinking, oversmoking, and carousing around and never exercising, except possibly in occasional violent weekend spurts. Will all this shorten your life? Yes, very likely more than diabetes will.

We can't offer any guarantees, but as Dr. Oscar Crofford of Vanderbilt University pointed out at the 1980 American Diabetes Association annual meeting, we already know that poorest control of diabetes is associated with highest risk of complications, while near-perfect control is associated with the lowest risk. So if you follow the recommended diabetic lifestyle, keep your blood sugar in good control, and keep your risks down, it is our unshakable belief that you can bring your span of years up to and even beyond that of the average person who is either unaware of the principles of good health or disinterested in following them.

A concrete testimonial to our theory is that over 850 people have been awarded the Fifty Year Duration of Diabetes medal by the Joslin Diabetes Foundation in Boston. The medal is given to people who have successfully lived fifty years or longer as insulin-dependent diabetics. This is a considerable achievement, because many people who earned the medal got diabetes before insulin was available. This means their early years with diabetes were particularly dangerous and detrimental. These people are the true heroes and heroines of diabetes. And there would be many, many more medal winners except that the Joslin Foundation requires complete medical records. There are also a large number of potential winners who haven't bothered to apply for the medal.

Naturally, if you ignore your diabetes and the good health principles it requires you to follow, you can make all the depressing statistics come true. So the real question is, Will *I* shorten my life? And only you can answer that one by the way you follow the diabetic program of diet and exercise.

How can I avoid the complications of diabetes?

We have mixed emotions about ranting at you about diabetes complications. Some doctors and nurses feel that unless they paint vivid horror pictures, diabetics won't take their disease seriously and do what they should to take care of it.

Sometimes this backfires, though, as we learned in a letter from one diabetic. On the first day of her diagnosis and hospitalization, she was told by the head nurse, "You have a dreadful, dreadful, dreadful disease." The nurse convinced her that all she had to look forward to was "becoming a blind, bilateral amputee, carried off to dialysis three times a week." This experience so affected her psychologically, she wrote, that

> I lay awake night after night shaken with an unbearable fear. It permeated every aspect of my daily life. I gave up wearing contact

lenses because I cried so much. I was worn out emotionally. My college doctor suggested psychiatric counseling. I was hesitant, but after six months I was helped greatly and started taking better care of myself because I finally felt there was a glimmer of hope for the future.

On the other hand, we can't just ignore or gloss over the complications. They can happen, but you have it in your power to make them *not* happen by keeping your diabetes under control— that is to say, keeping your blood sugar normal most of the time.

People intimately involved with diabetes either as patients or as health professionals have long believed that it's possible to avoid complications, especially since the new therapies of the last six to eight years started making high blood sugar controllable. Now their anecdotal evidence and gut feelings have finally been validated by science.

For example, the February 24, 1989, issue of the *Journal of the American Medical Association* published a detailed study of 230 diabetics in which the conclusions supported the idea that keeping your blood sugar normal is a way to avoid several of the major complications. In this study, no diabetic whose blood sugar was consistently less than 1.1 times normal had any of the expected eye and kidney problems of diabetes. In contrast, among those whose blood sugar was consistently greater than 1.5 times normal, 37 percent had eye problems (retinopathy) and 29 percent had kidney problems (beginnings of nephropathy).

In one of our SugarFree Centers we had the conclusions of the part of this study relating to eye problems confirmed months before the study appeared. We had invited an ophthalmologist to do a series of eye screenings for our clients. He had done his original work in diabetes at Los Angeles County–USC Medical Center, where practically every long-term diabetic had more or less severe retinopathy. This experience led him to believe that some degree of retinopathy was inevitable for diabetics. But when he tested our highly motivated, frequently blood-sugar-testing, multiple-injection-taking people, he found virtually no eye damage, and he has now completely reversed his original position.

So do everything in your power to keep your blood sugar normal. It's well worth the effort and then some.

How do I keep my blood sugar normal?

You asked the question correctly: "How do *I* keep my blood sugar normal?" Because diabetes is the original do-it-yourself disease. Although you'll have help and guidance from the health professionals on your diabetes team, the responsibility for day-to-day therapy is all yours.

Normalizing blood sugar involves many aspects of your life and lifestyle. You need a good diet, preferably one tailored to your needs by a dietitian, a sound exercise plan that you can stick to, some stress-control techniques that appeal to you and work for you, and self-education with magazines, books, and lectures to keep your knowledge growing. That will about do it for the great majority of you. Some Type II people will need to take pills, and some will need insulin. All Type I people will need insulin.

The more successful you are at these different aspects of self-care, the less you have to fear from diabetes and the more you have to gain in enhancing your total health. As Dr. Michael Bush of Cedars-Sinai Medical Center in Los Angeles, says, "This is one disease where *prevention* is far more possible than *reversal.*" So the greater dedication you have to managing your blood sugar, the greater will be your reward in feeling good and avoiding health problems associated with diabetes.

As to the question of what normal blood sugar is, the normal range is around 60 to 140 milligrams of sugar per deciliter of blood. The objective of all diabetes treatment is to keep blood sugar within this range.

After you eat, your blood sugar rises and reaches its peak between a half hour and one hour later. In nondiabetics it rarely goes over 150. Blood sugars above 160 suggest that a person is diabetic. Here is the normal pattern of blood sugar for nondiabetics in relationship to meals:

Relation to Food	Blood-Sugar Range
Fasting (before breakfast)	60 – 100
1 hour after meal	100 – 140
2 hours after meal	80 – 120
3 hours after meal	60 – 100

Diana Guthrie, a professor of nursing at the University of Kansas School of Medicine in Wichita, has provided us with this chart of recommended blood sugars for diabetics.

Relation to Food	Ideal	Acceptable
Fasting	80 – 110	120
1 hour after meal	100 – 150	180
2 hours after meal	80 – 130	150
3 hours after meal	80 – 110	130

You'll notice that on these charts the blood sugars you should aim for have both a lower boundary and an upper one. Although diabetes is primarily associated with blood sugars that are too high, insulin-taking diabetics often run the risk of having blood sugar that is too low. Low blood sugar, known as hypoglycemia, can result from too much insulin, too little food, too much exercise, etc. We will go into the details of hypoglycemia in the section for insulin-dependent diabetics. Type II diabetics who take pills can sometimes experience hypoglycemia, but it is milder and less frequent. We'll discuss that in the section for Type II diabetics.

Can anything besides eating and not eating make my blood sugar go up or down?

Yes, and you need to take these factors into account. Blood sugar often goes up when you have an infection—the flu, the common cold, stomach upsets. Major surgery and pregnancy cause a rise. Then there are a number of drugs that tend to raise blood sugar: caffeine, oral contraceptives, estrogen, and cortisone are the most important to know about. Emotional tension also causes blood sugar to swing upward.

Besides being lowered by fasting or by insufficient food, blood sugar goes down when you exercise strenuously. Among drugs with a lowering effect are alcohol (when you don't eat while drinking), large doses of aspirin, blood-thinning drugs, barbiturates, and sulfonamides.

For a complete list of medications that increase or lower blood-sugar levels, see the Reference Section: Medications that increase or lower blood-glucose levels.

How will I know if my therapy is working?

You take tests. Most of your testing will be self-testing. In a sense, you are your own laboratory technician. Here are the tests you will learn to perform.

Blood-sugar test. Your most important and most frequent test is a blood-sugar test. Only by testing your own blood sugar can you tell from day to day how well your therapy is working. And only if you make a record of your test results can your doctor see how good your control is or what modifications in your treatment are needed to improve it.

Thanks to modern technology, self-blood-sugar testing is now simple to learn and easy to do. And it's fast. Your results are available in between thirty seconds and two minutes, depending on the system you're using. Blood-sugar testing is performed by putting a small drop of your blood on a chemically treated pad.

Then you compare the color that the pad turns to a color chart (the less expensive method) or you use an electronic meter to interpret the blood sugar from the pad and give you a digital readout. This is more expensive but more accurate. Some of the newer meters use an electronic sensor rather than a chemically treated pad.

Most diabetes health professionals consider the development of self-blood-sugar testing to be the greatest advance in diabetes treatment since the discovery of insulin in 1922. Everyone should take advantage of it.

Type I diabetics who want to be in good control and who adjust their insulin dosage according to their blood sugar often take as many as four to seven blood-sugar tests a day. Type II's, once their blood-sugar levels have been normalized, can often maintain control with just three or four tests per week, backed up by an occasional four to six a day to see what the daily pattern looks like.

Hemoglobin A₁C test. Another test for assessment of control that all diabetics should use is the hemoglobin A_1C test, also called the glycosylated hemoglobin test. This test, combined with daily blood-sugar readings, gives you a total picture of your diabetes control, as it provides you with the long-range view.

The A_1C test analyzes how much glucose has bonded with red blood cells; this measurement indicates what your average blood sugar has been for the past two months. An A_1C test should be taken about every three months.

Ordinarily the A_1C is taken in a doctor's office, but there is now a test available for home use. It's called Self-Assure and is made by Evalulab (Drawer 1679, Palm City, Florida 34990; also available from the SugarFree Center for about $18). You put two drops of blood on the pad provided and mail it to the lab. Within two weeks you have the result, which can be sent either to your doctor or to you. If you have it sent to yourself, you should take it to your doctor for evaluation. Of course, if your results fall in the normal range, follow-up may not be essential.

Urine test. Before blood-sugar testing came on the scene, urine testing was the only way we had to know how well our diabetes was being controlled on a day-to-day basis. When blood sugar goes too far above normal, usually 150 to 180, some of the sugar spills over into the urine so that the body can get rid of it. Measuring the amount of sugar in your urine was supposed to indicate your blood-sugar level, but it was very inaccurate because:

- It indicated only what your blood sugar had been, not what your blood sugar was at the time of test;
- it couldn't tell you if your blood sugar was too low (hypoglycemia);
- it could be affected by such things as the amount of water you'd been drinking and any vitamins you'd been taking; and
- not everyone spills sugar when their blood sugar is between 150 and 180. Older people often don't spill until it's much higher (June doesn't spill until she's over 220), and children can show sugar in their urine when it's lower than 150.

So our advice is to forget urine testing except when you need to test for ketones.

Ketone test. You'll remember that ketones are the substances that accumulate in the blood and subsequently in the urine when glucose can't get into the cells and you burn your own fat and muscles for fuel instead of the carbohydrates you eat, which are normally the body's fuel.

Years ago there was a fad diet that had people eating only protein and fat (no carbohydrate). They were to test their urine for ketones every day and to be happy when they found ketones in it, because it meant they were burning fat and therefore losing weight.

Diabetics should *not* be happy to find ketones in their urine. In fact, if you find them, you should contact your doctor immediately for advice on how to get rid of them because their presence means you are seriously out of control.

How do I test for ketones?

A better question might be, *When* do I test for ketones? The answer for Type I diabetics is whenever two consecutive blood-sugar tests are over 200. For Type II diabetics who still produce insulin of their own, the situation is not so crucial, but all diabetics need to watch for ketones when they have infections, illnesses, or out-of-the-ordinary emotional stress.

The brand-name products to use for urinary ketone tests are Chemstrips K and Ketostix. You can also test for ketones using Chemstrips uGK and Keto-Diastix, which measure sugar in the urine as well.

What's the most accurate blood-sugar meter?

That's a question we hear virtually every day at our SugarFree Centers. It's a little awkward to answer because, as is often the case, the answer sounds vague. The reason is that 99 percent of meter accuracy depends on the operator. So the answer has to be that it's the one you can operate most accurately.

In truth, they *all* really work. The FDA must approve a meter before it's released to the public and won't let meters appear on the market if they're inherently inaccurate. They're all tested extensively. You can find the results of the required laboratory tests somewhere in each company's operator's manual or in their strip insert, usually under a heading like "Performance Characteristics." Here you can read all the statistical gobbledygook (correlation coefficient, range of coefficient variations, standard deviation, etc.) that proves the meter to have acceptable accuracy.

This leads to a corollary on the other side of the accuracy coin. When people report that a meter is inaccurate, what most of them should be saying is, "I can't operate this meter correctly" (or, if they really do know how to operate the meter correctly, "I don't like what this meter is saying about my blood sugar, so it must be wrong"). The technical-services department of one meter company reported that 90 percent of the meters returned to the company as reading inaccurately were operating perfectly.

How do I select the meter I can operate most accurately?

The first answer to this is easy: select the one your doctor or diabetes educator recommends. This is true for several reasons. It is usually the meter they use in their own office. It will therefore be easy for them to check out your meter (and your technique) any time you come into the office. Having the same meter as your health professional will give both of you confidence in the accuracy of your own test results. Health professionals have their prejudices, too. They often think the meter they have—and are most familiar with—is the only truly accurate meter.

Some doctors also have a machine that prints out your blood-sugar readings from a specific meter. In that case, they'd want you to have the meter that's compatible with their machine. Be sure you find out *exactly* which meter they recommend before you go shopping. Have them write down the name for you, because meter names are very similar and it's easy to get them confused.

If your health professional has no particular preference, you need to find the meter that's best suited to your lifestyle, economic situation, manual dexterity, visual acuity, blood volume, aesthetic taste, and whether the strips for the meter are covered by your health plan. To figure out all this, you'll need to read the brochures of all the meters or, better still, see all the meters in person and have someone knowledgeable explain the features of each. That's why you need to use as much care in selecting the place where you get your meter as you use in selecting the meter itself.

Where should I get my meter?

Let's start with some don'ts—the places where you *shouldn't* get your meter.

Don't get your meter by mail order. Although the Sugar-Free Centers have a mail-order service, we always say loud and clear, to anyone who will listen, that you should never order a meter by mail unless you have no other alternative. Since meter accuracy is so dependent on operator technique, it's absolutely vital that you receive thorough training and as much follow-up as you need as part of your meter purchase. You can't get that by mail order or by phone.

Don't get your meter from a place that has only one or two kinds of meters. If you have only a small selection, you're very unlikely to get the one that's just right for you. It would be like trying to put everyone into the same size shoe.

Don't get your meter from a "meter shover." As more and more meters enter the market and competition escalates, meter manufacturers, who once were very selective about where their meters could be sold and by whom, are now letting anybody and everybody sell their product. It may not be long before we even see meters stacked up at supermarket checkout stands or in corner vending machines.

At any rate, a meter shover is any outlet drugstore, discount house, etc.—that stocks meters but has neither the time nor the staff to teach you how to use them. All they do is shove your meter across the counter and say, "Here's your meter. The instructions are inside. That'll be . . ." No matter what price you

pay for a meter, if it is shoved at you with no instruction, you
have been grossly cheated.

Meter-shover horror story: Cathy Geer in our SugarFree
Center in San Bernardino, California, told us of a diabetic man
who came in for strips. He had just emerged from a week in the
hospital. How did he get there? He bought a meter over the
counter in a pharmacy without a lesson. He took it home, read
the instructions, listened to the tape that was included, and
started taking blood-sugar readings. They were almost all in the
normal range, so he felt very happy and confident. Then, when
he went to his doctor for his regular checkup, his blood sugar was
over 400 and he was showing ketones. The hospital was his next
stop. When Cathy analyzed his technique, she discovered that he
wasn't getting enough blood to cover the strip; hence the low
readings.

Don't let them "spiff" you. "Spiffing" is a cousin to the
old bait-and-switch technique. In retail parlance, it means pushing the product on which the biggest profit can be made. If a
salesperson tries to talk you out of a meter your health professional has recommended by claiming that another meter is much
better, you have cause to be suspicious.

To take a more positive approach: do get your meter from a
place with a large selection of meters, where you can sit down in
a quiet and caring atmosphere and receive expert advice and
meticulous instruction, a place where you can come back again
and again if you're confused and not be given the brush-off or
told something like, "Only Edna knows anything about these
meters, and she's not here."

It's a nice dividend if the place will also handle your insurance claims, but if your choice is between a place that gives good
instruction and doesn't make claims and a mail-order company or

meter shover that does, you're much better off choosing the instruction and making the claims yourself.

Once you've selected and purchased your testing supplies and equipment, you still have one remaining task: to learn the brand names of everything you use. Otherwise, on your first shopping trip to replenish your supplies you'll run into a lot of trouble. You may end up with the wrong product and not be able to return it if you opened it. And the brand names of all diabetes supplies are often similar. Believe it or not, we have many clients who come into our SugarFree Centers without knowing exactly what they want. Our advice is to bring in your empty container or write down the names of the supplies you need.

How do I get the drop of blood for my test?

In the early days of blood-sugar testing, diabetics had to stick themselves with an old insulin needle. Later they could do freelance jabbing with a lancet. Both ways were painful and ineffective. Now there are several excellent lancing devices that give you the right size drop of blood virtually painlessly. These include the Auto-Lancet, Autolet, Glucolet, Penlet, and Soft Touch.

There is also one little horror—the AutoClix. Fortunately it is no longer being manufactured, but there are still a lot of them floating around. This is because the makers of the device used to give it away in the hospital to newly diagnosed diabetics. Although that was a nice and generous idea, it backfired because the AutoClix was so painful that when people used it they often let out a loud *Aaaargh!* and promptly decided, "If this is what blood-sugar testing is like, I want no part of it." If you have an AutoClix, we want to assure you that this is definitely *not* what blood-sugar testing is like and urge you to rush out immediately and get one of the devices listed above, any of which will encourage you to take the number of tests you need to keep your blood sugar normal.

What can I do if I have trouble getting enough blood for the test?

First, try to relax. When you're tense, your blood tends to leave your extremities and go to your body organs to prepare you for the flight-or-fight response. You can tell if you are relaxed if you have warm hands.

Then make sure you're using the correct tip for your lancing device. Some of them have a choice of tips, one with a larger opening that makes a little deeper penetration than the normal tip. If you've checked that out and still have trouble, try some (or all) of the following:

1. Wash your hands with soap and very warm water. Allow warm water to run over your hands and wrists for at least one full minute. (Be sure you dry your hands thoroughly before starting your test.) Incidentally, washing your hands is much preferable to cleaning with alcohol. Not only does alcohol, when used repeatedly, dry out your skin, but if it hasn't evaporated before you take your test it can change the reading you get—usually making it lower.

2. Let your hand hang loosely by your side and shake it for at least thirty seconds.

3. Keeping your hand below heart level, milk the palm of your hand all the way up to the fingertip. Make sure the fingertip turns pink.

4. Prick the meaty side of the finger—not too close to the cuticle but not directly in the center (pad) of the finger or at the very top of the fingertip.

5. Allow your finger to relax for three to four full seconds before trying to squeeze the blood out. When you're cut or stuck with a sharp object, the muscles tighten up to prevent the release of blood. After a few seconds they relax and the blood flows easily again.

6. Milk your finger starting with the base on the palm side and working all the way up to the fingertip. Wait two or three seconds between milkings.

Where can you get blood for a test when you can't or don't want to use your fingertips?

We had a client who had received severe burns on both hands, including the fingertips, and needed to know if other areas of the body were possible sources for a drop of blood. We turned the question over to a doctor who always has original and innovative ideas. He didn't let us down. His answer, partially in jest, was that for your source of capillary blood you can use earlobes, penis (ouch!), or toes. (Venous blood is not the best to use because it doesn't have enough oxygen to react properly with the reagent strip.) However, before using toes, you must have your physician check your circulation with a Dopler blood-pressure study. If the value is 70 percent of that which is found in the arm, it is okay to use the toes for puncture. He also said the person should use a meter that does not require a great deal of blood.

Not long after this question came to us, we heard a talk by Dr. Peter Forsham. He told the story of a patient who was a concert pianist and obviously didn't want to use his fingers for the numerous tests he needed to take each day. His previous doctor had told him he'd just better find a new career. Dr. Forsham had a better plan. He asked the pianist which finger he used the least in his concerts. It was the one next to the smallest finger on the right hand. "Fine!" said Dr. Forsham. "Always take your blood sample from that same finger and always from the identical spot on the finger." Dr. Forsham explained that a benign tumor will develop on the spot from which you always take the blood. (We prefer to think of it as a callus.) You can continue to take blood from there, and it's just as good as from anywhere else and even hurts less. Problem solved. Pianist's career saved.

How do I keep a record of my blood-sugar readings?

It's great that you realize you should keep track of your blood-sugar readings. Blood-sugar testing is not an end in itself. You don't just test your blood sugar, look at the result, and say, "Nice test, there" or "Rotten test there," and go about your business. The results of your tests are important information to give health professionals so that they can analyze and evaluate them to see if your control can be improved. If you don't keep accurate records, they can't do the best job for you. The records are also valuable to you in seeing patterns in control—and lack of control.

Many meters now have memories ranging from one test all the way up to 334. But even if you're using a meter with a memory, you need to write out your test results in chart form so they can be quickly viewed. You can enter them in one of the many inexpensive log books currently available. A particularly good way to record the results is on GlucograF™ sheets developed by Dr. Richard K. Bernstein for use with his book *Diabetes: The GlucograF™ Method of Normalizing Blood Sugar.* With these sheets, you make dots on a graph for your blood-sugar readings, connect them with lines, and have an easy-to-read chart of your ups, downs, and normals. The sheets also have space to record such information as your insulin or pill dosage, meals, exercise, etc.—all the things that significantly influence your blood-sugar readings.

As we advance into the computer age, blood-sugar-testing technology is moving ahead with sophisticated data-management systems to coordinate with meters. Your doctor's office or the center from which you purchase your meter may have such a system, in which case it can run off your blood-sugar records for you. Or if you're really into computers, you may want to get your own system. If you have access to one of these data-management systems, remember that this will influence your meter selection, since most systems work only with the meter made by the same company. You can get information on these systems from your diabetes center or from a pharmacy offering a full line of diabetes equipment and supplies. You can also contact the companies themselves for information:

Ames (Glucofacts Data Management System), Miles, Inc., Diagnostics Division, Box 70, Elkhart, Indiana 46515, 800-348-8100.

Boehringer-Mannheim (Merlin Diabetes Management System), 9115 Hague Road, Box 50100, Indianapolis, Indiana 46250, 800-428-5074.

Diva Medical Systems (Romeo System), Riverplace, Suite 14, 10 Second Street, N.E., Minneapolis, Minnesota 55413, 612-623-9500.

Lifescan (Data Manager), 1051 Milpitas Boulevard, Milpitas, California 95035, 800-227-8862.

How can I learn more about taking care of my diabetes?

Read books. Read periodicals like *Diabetes Forecast, Diabetes in the News, Diabetes Self-Management* and, if you have a scientific turn of mind, *Diabetes* and *Diabetes Care* (see Recommended Reading).

Join your local affiliate of the American Diabetes Association (see Reference Section: Directory of Organizations) and attend their meetings. They usually have guest speakers— podiatrists, dietitians, ophthalmologists, or other professionals— who can fill you in on their own areas of expertise and answer questions that may have been puzzling you. Diabetes associations often sponsor day-long seminars with different speakers, panel discussions, and workshops. These are a terrific way to get a lot of diabetes information in a short period of time.

Find a diabetes education program in your area. Ask the ADA for names and places or write to the American Association of Diabetes Educators (see Reference Section: Directory of Organizations). These education programs sometimes charge a nominal fee, but you always get a lot more than your money's worth.

Diabetes education programs can involve a one-week crash course or weekly meetings over a period of time. They can be inpatient programs for newly diagnosed diabetics in the hospital, but most are outpatient. They can involve large or small groups, or they can offer individual instruction. There may be a group of teachers (nurses, dietitians, psychologists, social workers, etc.) or there may be one diabetes educator who handles the whole course. As you can see, you can usually find a program to meet your needs, whatever those needs may be.

Some diabetics we know are starting to form their own discussion groups so they can share experiences and helpful information with one another. Your doctor or the ADA or a diabetes education program may be able to put you in touch with other diabetics who are interested in forming such a group. You'll especially want to join a group if you agree with diabetic author Dorothea Sims: "Loneliness is one of the hardest things about having diabetes." (See Recommended Reading.)

Speaking of discussion groups, a film that we particularly recommend is *Diabetes: Focus on Feelings.* It shows a discussion group led by diabetes educator and clinical-social-work consultant Noreen Hall Papatheodorou. This is a tremendously moving and revealing film that can crack the shell of the most resentful and intractable of diabetics and can give family members insights into a diabetic's feelings that might otherwise take years to pry out. Ms. Papatheodorou has written a discussion guide to go with the film, and both are available from Pyramid Films, Box 1048, Santa Monica, California 90406. You might write to them and ask if this film, or any of their other excellent films on diabetes, is scheduled for showing in your area. If not, you could get together with a group and rent it yourself.

Keep at your learning. It's not just a one-time thing. There are new things to learn every day, and the new things almost invariably improve your health and make your life as a diabetic easier to handle.

Where can I find out about the latest developments in diabetes therapy as soon as they happen?

You could read all the publications in the field of diabetes. That's a good way, but not the best or most efficient. A surer method is to keep track of the *business* of diabetes. Find stockbrokers who will send you a copy of the prospectus of any and all companies involved in diabetes research, equipment, and products.

For instance, we have a friend who's an account executive at a brokerage house. She recently sent us information on a company that was working on a noninvasive blood-sugar test. (That means one in which you don't have to stick your finger.) This company had just signed a contract with Johnson and Johnson (which owns Lifescan, the company that makes the One Touch Blood Glucose Monitoring System). So now we know that something we're all looking forward to is at least in the works.

Business journals and newspapers are another good source of information. As our stock-market friend said, "The *Wall Street Journal* is published every day, so it usually beats the *New England Journal of Medicine* in getting out medical news." She also sent us an article from *Investor's Daily* which told about a company that's working on a single-shot cure for diabetes using "cell transplantation." The company claimed it could have the product on the market in two years, but a spokesperson for the National Institutes of Health's diabetes program called this projection "rather optimistic." Nevertheless, the article went on to say that the company is "pressing ahead in hopes of tapping a potential $3-billion market."

And thereby hangs the tale of how developments in medical research generally come about. We don't want to discount altruism, but considering the growing number of diabetics, it's not too surprising that so many companies are entering the field with profit as a primary motive.

But however the developments occur, we'll be happy just as long as they do keep coming. So put out your antennae and you may soon be picking up the news we've all been waiting for—the news of a cure.

DIABETES AND YOUR EMOTIONS

How can I keep from being depressed over my diabetes?

It's not easy. It's only logical to be depressed when you first learn you have diabetes. And all the cheerful remarks people make about how much nicer it is to have diabetes than leprosy or than being run over by a moving van or some such nonsense do no good at all. You know that it's *not* better than having nothing wrong with you.

After all, you have to make many, many changes in your life, and at first glance these changes all seem to be for the bad. On top of that, you feel like an outcast. You're no longer like everyone else. Of course, no one ever *is* like everyone else, but at the moment you feel like the town pariah, and you're certain that all your friends are going to drop you now that you have diabetes.

You get the automatic "why me?" reaction. "Why should *I* be selected to get this rotten disease?" "Why should *I* be threatened with blindness or kidney failure or gangrene or an early death if I don't follow a rigid regime?" Why indeed? There's really no reason. It's just the breaks of the genetic game. As a doctor told us once at a meeting, "Every person carries around about forty-four genetic defects." One of yours happens to be diabetes, and the fact is that some people draw out far worse tickets than diabetes in the genetic lottery. But that doesn't make you feel any better. As A. E. Housman said, "Little is the luck I've had/and, oh, 'tis comfort small,/to think that many another lad/has had no luck at all."

So what do you do about all this? You can sit and resentfully mutter about cruel fate and wallow in your woe, or you can, as the old saying has it, take the lemon you were handed and make lemonade out of it. We read an article about a woman who is a successful author and consumer advocate on radio and TV in Los Angeles. She described her beginnings: "When we married, during the early years it was rough. We were poor, but I wasn't about to go on welfare. So I decided if I wanted clothes, I had to make them. If I wanted the best bread I'd better learn how to bake. What I did was take poverty and turn it into an art."

What you need to do is take diabetes and turn it into an art. Do all the things you need to do for your diabetes and make them enhancements to your life.

How do I turn diabetes into an art?

The beginning step is to accept the fact that you have diabetes. The first thing most people do with diabetes is to deny it. Oh, your mind may know you have diabetes, but everything else about you—your heart, innards, soul, imagination, all those things you really listen to—say, "This has nothing to do with me. I'll ignore it and it will go away."

Alas, it won't, and you'll never be able to practice the art of diabetes until you get rid of the idea you don't have it. As a matter of fact, you need to do more than just accept your diabetes. One young woman, after hearing us speak at a diabetes meeting, said to June, "You actually seem to embrace diabetes." That she does. Not that she wouldn't prefer not to have diabetes, but since she does have it, she's determined to squeeze all the good out of it she can.

What's good about having diabetes?

Without being ridiculously Pollyannaish about it, we can affirm that diabetes *does* do some positive things for you. This isn't just our idea. Many diabetics have written to us and told us about what they consider to be the advantages of diabetes.

For one thing, you learn the principles of good health. Until you're whammed with something dramatic like diabetes, you may just bumble along wrecking your health through bad habits, laziness, and ignorance. Diabetes teaches you the right way to live and gives you a reason for doing so. As one diabetic skier put it, "This disease, this condition will keep you healthy and fit for whatever your heart desires. I feel I'm better off because I'm not fat; never have I been out of shape, and I eat well and thoughtfully."

Diabetics often actually feel better than they did before having their disease. Young diabetics have reported to us that they do better in sports than their nondiabetic friends because they never eat junk food and always keep regular hours. They're in top-notch shape all the time. They also say they're less susceptible to the colds and flus that their friends pick up with seasonal regularity.

Diabetics often look better than their nondiabetic contemporaries. Conscientious diabetics are lean and vital, bright of eye and quick of step. People of the same age who don't have diabetes to goad them onto the path of healthful living are often pudgy, sallow, and lethargic.

Diabetes develops self-discipline. Young persons who have diabetes and must assume responsibility for their own care develop a mature attitude of self-sufficiency at an early age. The discipline of following the diabetic way of life carries over to school and work and sports and creative endeavors. It can help make you a successful person in all areas of living.

Sometimes diabetes even sparks ambition. We know a young diabetic woman who is a successful city attorney. She told us how her choice of a profession came about: "When I got diabetes in high school I knew I'd have it all the rest of my life. I realized it would be an expensive disease, and I decided I wanted to always be able to take care of myself—and take care of myself *well*—whether I ever got married or not. That's why I worked hard to prepare myself for a good career."

And having diabetes makes you more compassionate toward others with problems. You learn how to give help gracefully and receive help without embarrassment or resentment. This, after all, is what puts the humanity in human beings.

But perhaps best of all, diabetes makes you capable of change. To change is the hardest thing for people to do. That's why so many of us take the easy way out and stick in a rut for our entire lives, unable to rouse ourselves into action to make the changes that could make us into the persons we were meant to be.

Diabetes, because it requires changes, and rather dramatic changes at that, shows you that you *can* change. If you can change in one area, then you are capable of change in other areas. You can improve not only your health but your whole life.

How do I start making all the changes I have to for my diabetes?

Again, that's not a question with easy answers. Every time we go to a meeting of diabetes educators, the major topic is "Compliance." We don't really like this word because it sounds as if you should bend to the will of the doctor or nurse or dietitian who knows what's good for you, and you, you misbehaving rascal, refuse to comply. Actually, nobody can make you "comply," can force you to change your habits. That has to come from within. The late psychologist Abraham Maslow has explained that you can reach the point of change only after you pass through several emotional stages in a "hierarchy of needs."

First, you have to have your basic physiological needs met.

That is, you must have food to eat and a place to stay. We'll presume you have that. Then you have to feel safe. This one's often a problem when you're first diagnosed because, far from feeling safe, you feel threatened. When you've conquered that fear, you need to have feelings of belonging and love from others. Many times the love and belonging are there, but newly diagnosed diabetics don't realize it. They think that friends and family members will reject them because of their "flaw." After you recognize how wrong you were there, you need to develop or redevelop your feelings of self-esteem and self-love, realizing you're a good person who is worth taking care of, worth going to the trouble of *changing* for the better. Only when you reach that point can you make those difficult changes.

Let's take you back to step two, the place where you feel threatened, unsafe, and afraid. Most, if not all, of your fear is fear of the unknown. Although people may have been throwing a lot of miscellaneous diabetes information at you, you probably haven't caught a tenth of it. Go back to the diabetes basics. As you learn them—really learn them this time, especially that diabetes is totally controllable—your fears should gradually dissolve. Without fear clouding your vision, we think you'll be able to see you haven't been abandoned and will become ready to accept the love that's all around you. You'll begin liking yourself—diabetes and all—and, lo, you may find that the needed changes in your life almost start making themselves.

But so much of the change seems to be giving up pleasures. How can I feel good about that?

We found that when June, in her early fits of depression, was ticking off all the pleasures she'd have to give up because of diabetes, what she was really ticking off were habits. Something like eating a sweet dessert was a habit that she considered a pleasure merely because she'd done it so often that it was a comforting part of her daily routine. The trick is to establish new *good* habits and turn them by constant use into pleasures.

This is not as hard as you may think. Eating a delectable, juicy piece of fresh fruit can become as much of a habit-pleasure as eating a big, gloppy dessert. For many people a daily bike ride or after-dinner walk is a pleasurable habit, and it can become one for you, too.

Furthermore, when you're thinking of the things you have to give up because of diabetes, think of these: you have to give up ever waking up with a hangover, either of the cigarette or alcohol variety; you have to give up discovering on a shopping trip that you've ballooned another dress or suit size; and you have to give up feeling and looking like a couch potato because of lack of exercise.

Finally, if, as you make the changes in your life, you still have moments of depression, try to keep in mind that it's part of the human condition to be depressed from time to time. There will be a natural tendency for you to lay your every woe on the doorstep of your diabetes. That's unfair to diabetes. Bad though it may be, it's not enough of a villain to be responsible for every dismal moment in your life. Even if you didn't have diabetes, you wouldn't be frisking around in a constant state of ecstasy. Though they call life the human comedy, it isn't all laughs for anybody.

But it isn't all tears, either, and you should make every effort to emphasize the good aspects of your life—to make yourself into a happy person.

How do I make myself happy?

You just do it. As Mark Twain said, "Everyone is just about as happy as he makes up his mind to be." And Robert Louis Stevenson believed that "there is no duty we so much underrate as the duty of being happy." So make up your mind and do your duty. It's vital that you do so for an important reason.

Not that you need a reason to justify happiness. It's a perfectly wonderful end in itself. But the reason we have in mind has only recently come to light. Studies reported in the *New York Times* show that being a happy, good-natured person can make you healthier, and that being an angry, suspicious person can be literally lethal: "People who are chronically hostile, who see the world through a lens of suspicion and cynicism, are particularly vulnerable to heart disease."

But that's not all. According to Dr. Ray H. Rosenman, a cardiologist at the SRI International Research Institute, hostile people are more prone to die prematurely from *all* causes, including cancer. They even get minor ailments like colds and the flu more often than happier people.

Your anger doesn't have to be the explosive, blow-your-top variety, either; more subtle styles of hostility—skepticism, mistrust, a tendency to make snide comments—are just as damaging. Strangely enough, even competitive, hard-driving type-A personalities who are not hostile are less at risk than their more antagonistic counterparts.

Try this experiment. The next time you feel hostile and angry, take you blood sugar. Assuming your negative feelings aren't due to low blood sugar, you'll probably discover your blood sugar ascending. Conversely, when you feel happy, take it and you may find, as June did once when she was looking forward to a trip to San Francisco, "I'm so happy I can't keep my blood sugar up."

Another reason to try to cut back on your anger is because of what it does to those around you. Many diabetics are angry because they have diabetes, but they don't like to admit the source of their anger, not even to themselves, so they displace their anger onto something or someone else. It could be the doctor's bill or the meter that gives a high blood-sugar reading or the health professional who's trying to help them make changes in their lives that they don't want to make or even their loving family members and friends.

The worst thing about displaced anger is that if you never admit its true source, you'll never get rid of it. It will keep festering within and erupting without. As the psychologist Willard Gaylin puts it, "Expressing anger is a form of public littering . . . how futile and dangerous it is."

Gaylin says that one cause of anger is a feeling that you don't have control of a situation. Since diabetics often feel out of control, both literally and figuratively, it's not too surprising that they're prone to anger. Working positively toward control over your diabetes and your emotions can diffuse anger.

David Burns, M.D., author of *Feeling Good,* believes that another source of anger is the feeling that a situation is unfair. And what could be more unfair than having diabetes? His book shows how to get rid of anger as well as other negative emotions like guilt and depression that cloud your existence and block out the sunshine of life.

Remember that happiness is good for what ails you—including diabetes. Try to take multiple shots of it every day.

How does getting emotionally upset affect my diabetes?

An emotional upset has about the same effect on blood sugar as chocolate-chip cookies. A fight with an intimate, a boost in rent, a week of final examinations—any stressful event in your life can send diabetes dramatically out of control. The strange thing is that even if something favorable takes place in your life, that, too, can sometimes raise blood sugar. When we were consultants on a tour to Hawaii for diabetics, several of the participants told us they got out of control with the excitement of packing for the trip.

Our own experience has convinced us that if you're working very hard at good control and usually achieve it but find that during certain periods there is a change for the worse and you can't figure out why, try getting out from under your normal life situation, especially if it's more hectic than usual. You may find, as June frequently does, that there's nothing wrong with your diabetes therapy, but that there *is* something wrong with your life and that *that's* what needs to be changed.

We are so convinced of the need for diabetics to learn how to handle the stresses of comtemporary life that we wrote an entire book on the theme. The revised edition of *The Diabetic's Total Health Book* explains why tensions and stresses have a negative effect on diabetes, what stressors you can avoid, and how to develop techniques to keep those you can't avoid from upsetting your control. A good portion of that book is devoted to instruction in relaxation therapies. These therapies—exercise, self-hypnosis, biofeedback, meditation, and guided imagery—are the best preventive medicine ever invented. Each of you should start practicing the ones that appeal to you most. You'll particularly enjoy practicing our unique all-purpose relaxers: laughter, travel, pets, and hugs, all of which will enhance your life and the lives of all those around you. *The Diabetic's Total Health Book* is published by Jeremy P. Tarcher. If you can't find it at your bookstore, write to us at the SugarFree Centers.

DIABETES AND YOUR DIET

What is the diabetic diet?

You hear a lot of talk about "the diabetic diet," and we ourselves sometimes fall into the trap of using that term. In reality, though, there is no one diabetic diet.

In the first place, the general diabetic diet is not a diet in the way most people think of one—a rigid and unnatural eating pattern that you follow until you remove extra pounds, at which time you revert to your old way of eating (and almost invariably put the pounds back on again). It's more a lifelong eating plan that should do three things for you:

Keep your diabetes under control. Your diet is of primary importance in controlling your blood sugar. For good control, Type I diabetics should focus on counting carbohydrates, since carbohydrates are primarily what is converted into glucose, which raises your blood sugar. Type II's should count calories, since calories add weight and many Type II's have a weight problem that makes it difficult for them to control their blood sugar.

Keep you healthy. Important as it is to keep your diabetes under control, that's not enough. You're much more than just a case of diabetes. You're a whole living person, not just a pancreas, and you need to eat a healthy diet for that whole living person. We're alway amused to see those exchange lists for fast-food establishments that make it look as if you could follow the exchanges, eat fast food for every meal, and live healthily ever after. You can't. You need to follow the general principles of dietary health, just as everyone else interested in longevity and feeling good does.

Let you enjoy your meals. Your food should be a pleasure—even a joy—and not some kind of grim health ordeal. That's one of the reasons we suggest you consult a dietitian; by doing that, your individual diabetes diet can be adjusted to your taste rather than vice versa. Otherwise, not only will your meals be unpleasant, but there's no possibility that you'll stick to the eating plan very long.

The American Diabetes Association and the American Dietetic Association now recommend that diabetics eat, on a per-meal basis, a diet of 55 to 60 percent carbohydrate, 12 to 20 percent protein, and 20 to 30 percent fat. (All foods are composed of various combinations of carbohydrate, protein, and fat.) These are the same proportions of nutrients that are recommended as health enhancing for all Americans. Most of us are still overeating both protein and fat. Some people's diets are as high as 40 percent fat, and most of that fat is the worst kind—saturated or animal fat, which causes high cholesterol. For diabetics, a particular worry is that it can make insulin less effective.

The American Diabetes Association's booklet *Exchange*

Lists for Meal Planning (available for $1.95 from the ADA or from the SugarFree Centers) is designed to help you, working with your dietitian or doctor, plan a daily diet so that each of your meals has approximately the same number of calories and the correct amount of carbohydrate, protein, and fat. The ADA exchange lists group together foods that are alike. There are six food-category lists from which you choose: starch/bread, meat and meat substitutes, vegetables, fruits, milk and milk products, and fats. You are assigned a certain number of choices (exchanges) from each list for each meal. So it becomes easy to plan meals of great variety but similar nutritional content.

The lists also indicate which food choices are high in sodium, fat, or fiber. Sodium and fat should be limited. Fiber should be increased, because it helps slow down the effects of foods that might otherwise send blood sugar soaring. There is a special *Exchange Lists for Weight Management* for people needing to lose weight. In addition, there are three supplements for special dietary problems: *Guidelines for Use of the Exchange Lists for Lowfat Meal Plannning, Guidelines for Use of the Exchange Lists for Low-Sodium Meal Planning,* and a combination of the two, *Guidelines for Use of the Exchange Lists for Low-Sodium, Lowfat Meal Planning.*

An alternative diet especially beneficial for Type II diabetics is the one created by Dr. James Anderson of the Veteran's Administration hospital in Lexington, Kentucky. Dr. Anderson was the original champion of oat bran in this country. His plan, the High Carbohydrate Fiber (HCF) nutrition plan, is helpful for overweight non-insulin-dependent diabetics. It can lower insulin requirements and eliminate the need for pills in many Type II diabetics. (For books explaining this diet, see Recommended Reading.)

A diet plan designed especially for lean, hard-to-control Type I (insulin-dependent) diabetics who produce little or no insulin of their own is favored by Dr. Richard K. Bernstein of Mamaroneck, New York. His book *Diabetes: The Glucograf*™

Method for Normalizing Blood Sugar explains this diet, which consists of 15 percent carbohydrate, 45 percent protein, and 40 percent fat. Dr. Bernstein himself has had diabetes for forty-two years, and this is the diet he created for control of his own diabetes.

Dr. Lois Jovanovic-Peterson, who coauthored *The Diabetic Woman* with us, thinks that dietary recommendations should always be based on a person's type of diabetes. In her opinion, the ideal diet for one type of diabetes may worsen control in another type. She points out that the goal of diet is to help maintain normal blood sugar, so the ideal diet for each person is the one that facilitates keeping that person's blood sugar normal. Thus diets must be individualized. Only your blood-sugar tests can tell you if your diet is working.

For all these reasons and because there are so many dietary options, we think working with a dietitian is the best way to find the eating plan that is right for you.

How can I find a dietitian?

If there isn't one on your doctor's staff, ask for a recommendation or call the local hospital and ask for a recommendation.

You might also get in touch with the local affiliate or chapter of the American Diabetes Association, or write to the American Dietetic Association for a list of names of dietitians in your area. You could also contact the American Association of Diabetes Educators. Many members of this organization are dietitians with a particular interest and expertise in diabetes. (See Reference Section: Directory of Organizations.)

Sometimes dietitians are listed in the yellow pages of the telephone directory. They may be listed under "Nutritionists" as well. But you have to be careful. There are some strange types who call themselves nutritionists and may try to put you on seaweed and soybeans and promise you the moon (that is to say, a cure). Stay away from these at all costs (and their costs are likely to be high; the moon is an expensive commodity).

Make sure the dietitian is an R.D.—a registered dietitian. And try to find one who has enough imagination and knowledge to open up meal possibilities geared to your own tastes and needs and not one who just gives the same food prescription to all diabetics.

How do I find out how many calories a day I should be consuming?

Again, the best way is to consult your dietitian, who will assign you the correct number of calories to eat. Sometimes your doctor is the one who does this for you. The Joslin Clinic in Boston has a neat formula by which you can work out the number of calories you need if you know what your weight should be (see Recommended Reading). Relatively inactive people should eat eleven calories per pound of body weight a day. Active people need around fourteen calories per pound. To lose weight, the clinic recommends eating less than eleven calories per pound a day— ideally, about nine. To gain weight, eat more than eleven calories per pound each day, say between fourteen and sixteen.

Also, you have to remember that men can eat more calories than women and that growing children and adolescents use more energy and need more food than adults or older people. We once read a rule of thumb that after the age of forty, people need about 10 percent fewer calories each decade if they want to stay the same weight. That's exactly the kind of information we all hate to hear, but it does have validity in nutritional circles.

Table 1 can used as a general guideline.

How can I make myself follow the diabetes diet?

You can conjure up horror stories in your imagination about the terrible things that will happen to you if you don't. But a strong

Median Body Weight of Men		Daily Calorie Allowances According to Age		
1b	*kg*	*22*	*45*	*65*
110	50	2200	2000	1850
121	55	2350	2150	1950
132	60	2500	2300	2100
143	65	2650	2400	2200
154	70	2800	2600	2400
165	75	2950	2700	2500
176	80	3050	2800	2600
187	85	3200	2950	2700
198	90	3350	3100	2800
209	95	3500	3200	2900
220	100	3700	3400	3100

Median Body Weight of Women		Daily Calorie Allowances According to Age		
1b	*kg*	*22*	*45*	*65*
88	40	1550	1450	1300
99	45	1700	1550	1450
110	50	1800	1650	1500
121	55	1950	1800	1650
128	58	2000	1850	1700
132	60	2050	1900	1700
143	65	2200	2000	1850
154	70	2300	2100	1950

Data from Food and Nutrition Board, National Academy of Sciences, National Research Council: Recommended dietary allowances, ed. 8, Washington, D.C., 1974, U.S. Government Printing Office, p. 29.

TABLE I. Calorie allowance for adults for various body weights and ages, assuming light physical activity.

positive approach is better. Make your meals so delicious and interesting that you *want* to follow your diet. Make your eating not a grim therapy, but a pleasurable delight. There are lots of gourmet cookbooks available for diabetics (see Recommended Reading). Try new recipes. Try variations on old recipes. Try different herbs and spices (most of these are free, diabetically speaking). And don't overlook the aesthetics of food serving. A few flowers on the table give you no extra carbohydrates or calories and do a lot toward making mealtimes a pleasure.

This all holds especially true if you live alone. June, in her prediabetic days, often used to have for dinner what we called an "avocado sandwich maybe," since whenever someone asked her what she was having for dinner, she usually responded vaguely, "Oh, I guess I'll have an avocado sandwich maybe." Which meant she had no idea what she was going to have and didn't intend to make any plans. She was going to grab whatever she found in the refrigerator, if anything.

Now June always has a well-planned and delicious meal that she eagerly looks forward to. Her appetite is also better. And strangely enough, although she's eating fewer calories, she's eating more—and more satisfying—food. This is because she's cut down on high-calorie fats and entirely cut out high- (and empty-) calorie junk foods.

The most ghastly diabetic diet idea we've ever heard of is the result of a man's decision that calculating the diabetic diet is too much of a chore. He resolved to eat the same breakfast, the same lunch, and the same dinner every day. Ugh! Besides being lethally boring, this is nutritionally unsound. Diabetics need a lot of variety in their diets in order to make certain they're covering all the nutritional waterfronts. Not only that, but, as a home economist told us wryly, "you should eat a great variety of foods because there are so many chemicals in everything these days, it's the only way you can avoid getting a big buildup of one chemical that might cause harmful side effects."

Which foods are best for keeping my blood sugar normal?

First, you have to realize that it is mainly the carbohydrates in foods that are converted directly into glucose and affect your blood sugar. True, about 65 percent of protein becomes glucose, but since it takes six or eight hours to do so, it has more of a stabilizing than an escalating effect. Fat is not changed to glucose—one of its few virtues for diabetics.

But all carbohydrates are not created equal. There was no scientific data on what effect individual carbohydrate foods have on blood sugar until 1983, when Dr. David Jenkins and fellow researchers at the University of Toronto published the Carbohydrate Glycemic Index (see Table 2). This is a classification of how high and how fast certain foods raise blood sugar. The problem with the index is that in compiling it only sixty-two foods were tested.

For diabetics, generally speaking, a food with a low (slow-releasing) glycemic index is preferred to one with a high (fast-releasing) index. The foods on the index are compared to glucose, which is assigned the top figure of 100. The findings are often surprising: sucrose (table sugar) is only 59, while carrots (cooked) are 92; instant potatoes are 80, but sweet potatoes are only 48. Ice cream is only 36, so index-wise it's as good for diabetics as lima beans, which are also 36. If you're thinking there must be a catch, there is. A bowl of ice cream has a lot more calories—and the wrong kind—than a bowl of lima beans. In other words, you cannot and should not eat by glycemic index alone. Blood sugar is not the only factor to consider; calories and nutritional values count, too.

It's also known that when carbohydrates are eaten as part of a meal that includes protein and fat rather than alone, blood sugar rises less. A further complication is that not all people respond to different kinds of carbohydrate in the same way. In a sense, you need to use your blood-sugar tests to figure out how

Simple Sugars

Fructose—20
Sucrose—59

Honey—87
Glucose—100

Fruits

Apples—39
Oranges—40
Orange Juice—46

Bananas—62
Raisins—64

Starchy Vegetables

Sweet Potatoes—48
Yams—51
Beets—64
White Potatoes—70

Instant Potatoes—80
Carrots—92
Parsnips—97

Dairy Products

Skim Milk—32
Whole Milk—34

Ice Cream—36
Yogurt—36

Legumes

Soybeans—15
Lentils—29
Kidney Beans—29
Black-eyed Peas—33

Garbanzos—36
Lima Beans—36
Baked Beans—40
Frozen Peas—51

Pasta, Corn, Rice, Bread

Whole-wheat Pasta—42
White Pasta—50
Sweet Corn—59
Brown Rice—66

White Bread—69
Whole-wheat Bread—72
White Rice—72

Breakfast Cereals

Oatmeal—49
All-Bran—51
Swiss Muesli—66

Shredded Wheat—67
Cornflakes—80

Miscellaneous

Peanuts—13
Sausages—28
Fish Sticks—38
Tomato Soup—38

Sponge Cake—46
Potato Chips—51
Mars Bars—68

TABLE 2. Carbohydrate Glycemic Index.

you respond to different foods. You need to create your own glycemic index.

Though there are these drawbacks to the glycemic index, we find that it is for many people a very helpful guide to foods likely to help or hinder control. Eating more of the foods with an index of 50 or lower and less of those with higher ratings might make an encouraging difference to many of you who have been innocently consuming too many foods at the top of the scale.

Do I have to measure my food?

Yes, it's the only way to be sure you're getting the amount of food your diet specifies, neither more nor less. *Exchange Lists for Meal Planning* gives portions in cups and tablespoons or teaspoons as well as in weight. Unfortunately, this sometimes leads to sizable variations in amounts, so you should stick to ounces and actually weighing. Type I people, especially, need to be careful to eat portions of the correct size in carbohydrates. This is where a food scale comes in handy.

Using bagels as an example, our science-trained friend Daisy Kuhn, a professor of microbiology, gave us a great lesson in carbohydrate variation in the starch/bread exchanges on the lists. Each serving on the starch/bread list is supposed to have about 15 grams of carbohydrate and eighty calories. For a bagel exchange, the list says "½ (1 oz.)" as the amount to eat. In actuality, not many half bagels are only one ounce (approximately 30 grams). To check on this figure, Daisy bought some bagels at a local deli. Using her Soehnle food scale, which gives weight in both ounces and grams, she found that a half bagel weighed 2¼ ounces, and therefore contained 33⅘ grams of carbohydrate. As a Type I diabetic she knew that if she hadn't weighed her bagel she would have eaten over twice the carbohydrate she wanted to and probably would have run up a high blood sugar. Type II's, of course, would be eating twice the calories they wanted to.

Likewise, a slice of bread should be limited to one ounce. But what a difference there is in reality between most supermarket bread and what you find in health-food stores or in bakeries. So get yourself a Soehnle or equivalent scale and do some weighing, at least at the beginning of your new eating plan. Or, even better, use the easy way to weigh food and convert it to exchanges—buy a Diabetic Exchange Center food scale. Manufactured by Health-O-Meter, a division of Continental Scale Corporation, it gives you the weight of your food in ounces and then converts this to food exchanges. It is available at the SugarFree Centers and at some diet centers.

If you're really conscientious at first about weighing and measuring your food, you'll be amazed at how quickly you learn to eye-measure or, as with bread, hand-weigh when you're out to dinner at a friend's house or in a restaurant. (Hint: sometimes it helps to discreetly nudge your food into little piles, the better to estimate the quantity.) You may get so good at eye-measuring and hand-weighing that you can do weight- and quantity-guessing parlor tricks, like the guy who guesses weights at the circus. Of course, the real and worthwhile trick is using your skill to eat the exact amount of food on your diet.

Can I save up food exchanges from one meal and use them for the next?

Definitely not. One of the most important principles of the diabetic eating plan is having every meal well balanced and eating neither more nor less than is called for. A diabetic, especially an insulin-dependent one, would really get into trouble following the great American eating pattern of nothing much for breakfast, a light lunch, and a gorging session at night. As a matter of fact, all those nondiabetics who do follow this scheme are getting themselves into trouble, too. They don't feel their best, they don't function well, and they're often putting on wads of fat.

The only exchange you can ever save up is your fat exchange. We don't mean that you can save fat exchanges for several days and then lap up a pint of whipping cream. It's more like saving one fat exchange from breakfast and one from lunch and using them at dinner. Even this shouldn't be a standard method of operating, only an occasional indulgence to be particularly avoided when an increase in activity is planned after a meal.

Is there anything I can eat all I want of without counting it in my diet?

You can hype up the flavors of your meals with herbs and spices without counting them. And you can eat as much of the following vegetables as you want, if you eat them raw: chicory; Chinese cabbage; endive; escarole; iceberg, butter, red-leaf, or romaine lettuce; parsley; and watercress. There is a list of such "free foods" in *Exchange Lists for Meal Planning.* You can also eat all the unsweetened rhubarb, unsweetened cranberries, and un-flavored gelatin that you can possibly hold. Yum!

Can a diabetic follow a vegetarian diet?

Of course. We consider the vegetarian diet extremely healthy for everyone and especially good for non-insulin-dependent diabetics who are overweight. In fact, Dr. James Anderson's HCF diet (see page 44) is as close as it can get to a vegetarian diet without being one.

One advantage of vegetarianism is that the diet is naturally low in fat and high in fiber. Many of the staples of the diet— soybeans, beans, oats, lentils, pasta, rice—are low on the Car-bohydrate Glycemic Index (see page 50). This, along with their high fiber content, means that food becomes glucose at a slow pace and blood sugar stays normal more easily. In addition to helping control diabetes, a vegetarian diet reduces the risk of heart disease and tends to promote weight loss.

There is more than one type of vegetarian diet: *vegan*, or no animal food at all; *lacto-vegetarian*, all vegetable except for milk, cheese, and other dairy products; and *lacto-ovo-vegetarian*, in which both dairy products and eggs can be eaten. The problem with vegan is that calcium and iron may be in low supply and a pill supplement may be advisable. The main problem with all vegetarian diets is that they can be deficient in vitamin B_{12}, which can be taken in pill form but is more effective when injected. So if you're an insulin taker and familiar with the injection process, you might ask your doctor about shooting your own B^{12}.

To follow a vegetarian diet as a diabetic, you need special food lists for guidance in calorie content and carbohydrate and fat amounts. The most complete lists we know of are in Marion Franz's *Exchanges for All Occasions.* Our favorite vegetarian cookbook is *The New Laurel's Kitchen*, which, unlike many such cookbooks, is not laden with sweets and fats. See Recommended Reading for a complete list of exchange lists and cookbooks.

Will I be able to follow my diet in restaurants?

Of course. It won't be as easy as following it at home, where you can select and measure everything to make sure you're getting exactly what you need, but with a little experience and ingenuity it can be done. In fact, it is done by diabetics every day.

At first, when you're just getting started with diabetes, you might want to check out the restaurant ahead of time to see what they have on the menu that would be right for you. This gives you time to figure out in advance what you want to order. You can also find out if they have, for example, fruit for dessert rather than something gloppy and sweet. If they don't, you can bring along a piece of fruit and either eat it there or eat it after you leave.

Checking out the restaurant ahead of time is also a good idea because you'll know if it's open. Sometimes on a trip June has gone out to a restaurant recommended in a travel book or article only to find it's been closed for six months. This can be more than an awkward situation if it's time to eat and there's no other restaurant around.

For insulin-dependent diabetics, a reservation is very important. The person taking the reservation should be informed that one of the diners is a diabetic, that the table *must* be ready at the time of the reservation, and that the food *must* be served without undue delay. (None of this sitting around in the bar for an hour waiting for a table, which happens in a lot of restaurants that may be trying to get you to buy extra drinks.)

What kinds of things should I order in restaurants?

As long as you avoid concentrated sweets, you can usually order anything you want. At first, though, try to avoid unfamiliar concoctions that are likely to have a lot of sauce (sauces often contain a great deal of carbohydrate and fat). Straightforward poultry or fish, and bread and vegetables are the easiest things to recognize and measure.

This doesn't mean you're forever stuck with plain fare. As you gain more experience, you'll be able to do more daring dining in ethnic restaurants. Actually, it won't be daring at all if you do a little cookbook research on various ethnic dishes. When you know what's in a dish—say *pasta e fagiole* or *blanquette de veau* or beef in oyster sauce—you'll know whether it's a good idea for you. In time you'll also learn to eye-measure your food and known how much of a certain dish you can eat.

What do you mean by concentrated sweets?

Concentrated sweets are what, when you taste them, are sweet, all sweet, and nothing but sweet. They're sugar, honey, and syrup. They're candy, frosted cake, pies, cookies, and ice-cream sundaes. They're almost everything listed on restaurant menus as desserts. They're all soft drinks, except artificially sweetened ones.

Concentrated sweets are an assault upon your system that

sends your blood sugar soaring. Besides that, they quickly use up
your daily allotment of calories without giving you any real food
value in return—empty calories, as they're known.

Are there any sweeteners I can safely use?

Sweets are a problem for most people—diabetic or not. We
seemed to be programmed to like them. It may be biological: our
ancestors had to have this craving for sweets to inspire them to
climb trees for fruit, which would give them the vitamins they
needed. Or it may be psychological, because we were rewarded
with sweet treats when we were good little girls and boys; it
showed we were approved of and loved, and we keep seeking this
easy access to love and approval. Or it may be a combination of
the two, which makes it even harder to kick the sweets habit.

There are some lucky souls who have no particular craving
for sweets. They can take them, but they can just as easily leave
them alone. June is one of these. She enjoys an occasional sweet
treat such as a little jam on her toast, but she could just as well
get along without it.

But for those of you for whom giving up sweets is a great
loss and deprivation, there are sweets that you can have *occasionally* and *if you count them in your diet.* But since none of these is
loaded with vitamins and minerals, you wouldn't want them to
take the place of the nutritious items you need.

There are two kinds of sweeteners: noncaloric and caloric.
The noncaloric sweeteners include saccharine, aspartame (NutraSweet and Equal), cyclamates, and Sunette (Sweet One). The
most commonly used caloric ones include sucrose (the dreaded
and ubiquitous sugar, which we won't talk about here), fructose,
sorbitol, mannitol, and HSH. Caloric sweeteners should not be
"ingested freely," as dietitians like to put it. We actually don't
feel that *any* sweetener should be ingested freely, since you never
know when a laboratory mouse is going to clutch his bladder or

liver and topple over and cause hysterical headlines about a previously approved sweetener. So again you have that good old boring admonition to practice moderation.

One way of achieving moderation is not to concentrate on one kind of sweetener but to vary them, never having more than a couple of items sweetened with any one kind of artificial sweetener a day. That way if the mouse topples, you won't have to worry that your system is loaded with lethals.

Following is a rundown of the various sweeteners and how to fit them into your diet.

Caloric Sweeteners

Fructose. There are several good things to say about fructose. First off, it's not an artificial sweetener. It is, as they like to say about almost every product you see in markets these days, "all natural." It is found in sweet fruit and most vegetables. It is also available in granular and liquid form in diabetes supply centers. It tastes sweet and has about the same calorie count as sugar (one hundred calories per ounce). But because it is much sweeter than sugar, you can use less of it to get the same sweet taste. The graph on page 58, reprinted from *Laurel's Kitchen*, shows how much sweeter it is.

Fructose also doesn't raise your blood sugar as fast or as high as sucrose. The Carbohydrate Glycemic Index (see p. 50) gives it a 20 as compared with a 59 for sucrose and a 100 for glucose. One caution: *if your blood sugar is already high, fructose will raise your blood sugar just as fast and as high as sugar.*

If you want to use fructose in baking, our former dietitian Ron Brown suggests that you use it for one-quarter of the sugar in the recipe and a noncaloric sweetener for another quarter. You can usually just leave out the rest, he says, since most desserts are too sweet anyway.

The British Diabetic Association reports that when you use fructose in cakes, it tends to keep them fresher longer and also

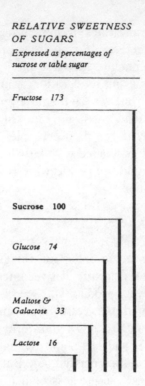

RELATIVE SWEETNESS
OF SUGARS
Expressed as percentages of
sucrose or table sugar

Fructose 173

Sucrose 100

Glucose 74

Maltose &
Galactose 33

Lactose 16

Reprinted by permission from *Laurel's Kitchen* by Laurel Robertson, Carol Flinders, and Bronwen Godfrey (Nilgiri Press, 1976).

has a better taste than ordinary sugar. The association does caution, however, in capital letters and boldface type: **FRUIT SUGAR IS NOT SUITABLE FOR THE OVERWEIGHT.**

There have been some reports that fructose raises triglycerides (the principal form of fat stored by the body). But Margaret A. Powers, in her *Handbook of Diabetes Nutritional Management,* says that only large intakes of fructose—two hundred to five hundred grams per day—cause a raise in triglycerides, while moderate amounts do not. To put that in perspective, five hundred grams per day would be the equivalent of 188 fructose-sweetened chocolate truffles.

The terms *fructose* and *fruit sugar* are used interchangeably. In England and Europe, fructose is usually made from fruit; in the United States, it is made from corn. Fructose and fruit sugar are chemically the same, although some people claim there is a difference in taste.

Sorbitol. Sorbitol, a sugar alcohol found in many plants, like fructose, doesn't cause the blood sugar to rise as rapidly as sugar because of the way it's metabolized. Sorbitol suffers a bad press for its tendency to have a laxative effect in certain susceptible people. (We think of that as nature's way of promoting moderation.) We've also heard people denigrate sorbitol as an artificial sweetener. Not true. Sorbitol is found naturally in fruit. It was our friend Daisy Kuhn, professor of microbiology at California State University at Northridge, who put us straight on this. She even gave June a basket of prunes and pears as a sorbitol Easter gift, explaining that these two fruits are among the highest in sorbitol. This, of course, explains why prunes work so well as a laxative. Other fruits with a high sorbitol content are plums, berries, apples, and cherries. Daisy tells us that it is safe for most adults to eat about 40 grams of sorbitol if it is spaced out over a day. A three-ounce serving of prunes has about 12 grams of sorbitol. Hard candies sweetened with sorbitol contain about 2.6 grams. Though many commercial foods are sweetened with sorbitol, consumers in the United States cannot buy it for home use.

Another erroneous bum rap for sorbitol is that it causes the diabetes complications of retinopathy and neuropathy. This is a confusion between two different sorbitols. The sorbitol that does the damage is a waste product produced from glucose in the bloodstream. It is definitely *not* the sorbitol eaten as food. (Incidentally, an enzyme called aldose reductase stimulates the conversion of blood glucose into sorbitol. For that reason a new drug is being developed to block the action of aldose reductase and thereby to prevent the development of these diabetes complications.) To reiterate: *sorbitol eaten as a food is not implicated in eye, nerve, or kidney damage.*

Mannitol. Mannitol, another sugar alcohol, is similar to sorbitol—including its laxitivity in susceptible individuals. It's also used as a commercial sweetening agent, although not as commonly as sorbitol.

HSH (Hydrogenated Starch Hydrolysate). Daisy Kuhn tells us that HSH is *chemically* the same as sorbitol. We've heard that it isn't quite as laxative as sorbitol, but since we've heard this mainly from companies that manufacture products made with HSH, we're waiting for more evidence to substantiate this claim. HSH is the sweetener in many sugar-free candies.

Noncaloric Sweeteners

People have very strong feelings about artificial sweeteners. Some won't touch them with a twelve-foot tongue. One woman called us in a fury to cancel her subscription to the *Health-O-Gram* because we mentioned Equal in it. And we once heard a lecture by a doctor, a medical adviser for an ADA chapter, in which he cited the many evils of saccharine, saying that it, and not cyclamates, should have been banned by the Food and Drug Administration. (He's been at least half vindicated, since the FDA has recently decided to lift its ban on cyclamates; by the time you read this they'll probably be back on the market.) By the way, any of the artificial sweeteners tasted alone will taste anywhere from bad to funny. They taste good only in foods and drinks. Here, then, is a brief rundown of the current crop of artificial sweeteners.

Saccharine. This is the primary sweetening component of Sweet 'N Low and Sugar Twin. It can be used in cooking. Some people find that it has a bitter or metallic aftertaste, but when combined with fructose in a recipe it's not noticeable. Because saccharine has been known to cause cancer when fed to animals in huge amounts, the FDA requires all products containing saccharine to bear the following warning: "Use of this product may be hazardous to your health. This product contains saccharine, which has been determined to cause cancer in laboratory animals." Those studies haven't yet been directly correlated to humans.

Aspartame (NutraSweet and Equal). This is currently the most popular noncaloric sweetener around—and it is around everywhere. It doesn't have the aftertaste of saccharine, but its tragic flaw is that it loses its sweetness in cooking or baking and doesn't have enough bulk for baked goods. One packet of Equal is equivalent in sweetness to two teaspoons of sugar. One tablet equals one teaspoon of sugar.

Since aspartame can be harmful to people with a rare metabolic abnormality called PKU (phenylketonuria), the FDA requires that it carry a warning on the package. The FDA considers that an acceptable amount of aspartame is up to fifty milligrams per kilogram (2.2 pounds) of body weight. Gloria Loring, in her *Kids, Food, and Diabetes*, translates this as one twelve-ounce can of aspartame-sweetened soda per 12 pounds of body weight. Actually, a 132-pound person would have to consume eighty-six packets a day to reach the FDA's maximum accepted intake.

Cyclamates. Until cyclamates are back on the market, we won't know the equivalences of the packages. We do know that a lot of people will be welcoming cyclamates back, especially those who've been doing their cyclamate runs to Canada during the years it has been banned in this country. People like the fact that is has no aftertaste and that you can cook with it.

Keep watching the newspaper for announcements of its return and the inevitable warning and praising articles that will appear in its wake. It is not yet known what kind of FDA warning it will have to bear—if any.

Sunette (Sweet One). Sunette was safely used outside the United States for five years before it was approved here. It's the only dietetic sweetener that doesn't require a warning label. (Apparently so far nary a mouse has toppled.) Sunette is two hundred times sweeter than sugar. Its big advantage is that it doesn't break down when heated; therefore, you can cook with it. Each packet gives the sweetness of two teaspoons of sugar, and each contains four calories and one gram of carbohydrate. The carbohydrate is in the form of dextrose. "Not to worry," says our dietitian Meg Gaekle. "It's added only to give bulk." (The manufacturers of Sweet 'N Low do the same thing.) In the small amounts generally used, it causes no problems.

A final reminder: honey, molasses, pure maple syrup, and other such sweeteners are not approved for diabetics no matter how many ill-informed health-food-store people tell you they are. For more information on sweeteners, see the Reference Section: How Sweet It Is.

What do I do if I am served too much food?

Leave what you can't eat or, in the case of expensive protein, take it home with you in a doggie bag. (You may have enough meat to last you for two or three meals.) June has the trick of carrying plastic bags in her purse and quietly bagging any excess.

One way to avoid getting plates that are bursting with calories is to go to restaurants that feature California or spa cuisine. But don't be sad if there aren't any of these in your area. They are usually very expensive, and you can actually sometimes get too little food in such establishments.

A happy trend in restaurant menus is the appearance of special "Pritikin Plates" and American Heart Association selections. These are low in calories and fat and high in fiber; watch for them. You should also watch for the restaurants that have special "light eater" dinners. There aren't many of these, but there are more and more all the time, because more and more people want to watch their weight or, as in the case of older people, just have diminished appetites.

Another possibility for getting smaller portions is to ask if you can have the children's dinner. Restaurants are sometimes willing to serve it to adults if you pay a small surcharge. It will still cost less than paying for the gross regular portions.

Our favorite trick for getting smaller portions and saving money and yet experiencing the best of dining out is to go for lunch rather than dinner. The portions are about half as large, with prices to match. A further advantage is that you're eating your main meal in the middle of the day, so you can walk it off afterward rather than just going to bed on a full stomach and letting it turn to fat. We especially do this main-meal-at-lunch trick when we travel. Dinner is then something light in the hotel coffee shop, or something we bring into the room.

Are salads always a safe bet when you're confused about what to order?

Let's take the ubiquitous salad bar, for example. It can be hazardous to your health in several ways. People sometimes cough and sneeze over salad bars, and to keep the ingredients fresh looking, they are often sprayed with allergy-causing sulfides. But worst of all, while you think you're restricting yourself to a diet meal, you're actually loading up on calories from the dressing. One study showed that the average person takes in more calories from a salad bar than he or she would from a standard meat-and-potatoes lunch.

It's not always that much better if the salad is brought to your table. As *Better Homes and Gardens* reported, a chef's salad with cheese, ham, turkey, and half an egg dolloped with blue-cheese dressing has seven hundred calories and fifty-eight grams of fat. For less than half the calories and 10 percent of the fat you can have a turkey sandwich made with two slices of whole-wheat bread, lettuce, and tomato.

Since dressing is the major culprit in a salad's assault on your diet, the only way to order salad is with dressing on the side. Then don't dump big globs onto your salad, but use this little trick a dieter once taught us: dip your fork into the salad dressing and then pick up the lettuce or other vegetable with the fork. Just enough dressing clings to the fork and is transported to the salad to give it flavor with minimal calories.

Can I eat in fast-food chains?

Yes, and you can eat from the pushcart of a Tijuana taco vendor, but neither would be the best choice for your overall health. As we mentioned previously, you can follow the diabetic exchange system and presumably keep your diabetes under control in fast-food chains, but the food there is far too high in fat (especially saturated fat—the wrong kind) and sodium and far too low in fiber. But we realize there is often no other choice for a quick and economical place to eat, and we also realize that for some high-school and college students fast food is a way of life. So when you must (or choose to) eat fast food, the following books are invaluable in helping you select what in horse-racing circles they call the best of a poor field:

Fast Food Facts, by Marian Franz, published by the International Diabetes Center, gives the calories, carbohydrate, protein, fat, sodium, and diabetes exchanges for the food served at twenty-six chains, including Arby's, Burger King, Chick-fil-A, Church's Fried Chicken, Dairy Queen, Domino's Pizza, Jack-in-the-Box, Kentucky Fried Chicken, Long John Silver's, McDonald's, Pizza Hut, Roy Rogers, Wendy's, Whataburger, and White Castle. There is a good introduction on the philosophy of dining in fast-food restaurants and the pitfalls to avoid. In the analysis of each restaurant's foods, there is a forthright list on foods not recommended.

The Fast Food Checker, published by Lite Styler, has the advantage of being pocket-sized so you can keep it with you at all times in case you suddenly find it necessary to eat in a fast-food place. It also has the advantage of listing, along with all the above information, the increasingly significant cholesterol content. Restaurants covered include Burger King, Carl's Jr., Domino's Pizza, El Pollo Loco, Hardee's, Little Caesar's Pizza, McDonald's, Subway, Taco Bell, Taco John's, Wendy's, and White Castle.

Another book, *The Diabetic's Brand Name Food Exchange Handbook,* published by Running Press, gives the calories, exchanges, and sodium content of four thousand supermarket products and the same information on foods served at most of the chains named above. But since this book doesn't include the fat and cholesterol content, it leaves you in the dark about two of the most significant health facts.

Being informed about the actual content of fast foods—along with the amount of fiber, which none of these books documents—is what should keep you out of most fast-food chains except on rare occasions.

We are happy to report that fast food is getting healthier. For example, the chicken at El Pollo Loco is low in fat and cholesterol, and while you couldn't call it low in sodium, it's a lot better on that score than most others. We actually think that healthy fast food is a commodity whose time has come. It's part of that diabeticization of America we talked about in the Introduction. People everywhere are getting more concerned about what they put into their bodies. When people want something—as they now want healthier fast foods and convenience foods in markets—the fast-food chains and food companies would be making an extremely poor business decision if they didn't start supplying them.

How can I stay on my diet when I'm invited out to dinner?

First, make sure that anyone who invites you to dinner knows you're a diabetic. That shouldn't be difficult, because people who know you well enough to extend the invitation will probably have long since been informed about your diabetes.

Almost anyone who knows you're a diabetic will ask what's special about your diet. An easy way to explain it is to show the person the answer to the question "How do I plan a meal for my diabetic friend?" (see the section "For Family and Friends"). If you don't have this book handy, just be sure to mention the piece of fruit for dessert. You might add that any vegetable is fine, except those high on the glycemic index, such as cooked carrots, parsnips, and beets.

When you're actually eating dinner, do just as you would at home or in a restaurant. That is, don't eat more than you should just to be polite. It's always sound policy to wildly praise the host's or hostess's cooking as you eat your way through everything you can, all the while expressing profound regret that you can't gobble up every morsel and even have second helpings. Your words will probably speak as loudly as your actions do, and the combination should indeed satisfy the most sensitive of cooks.

How do I make it through the holidays without breaking my diet?

Remember the origin of holiday festivals? They were the few occasions in the year when peasants who ran around most of the time with hollow, rumbling stomachs could really fill up. Now, however, most of the people in this country aren't perpetually hungry. On the contrary, what a biologist friend of ours calls "hyperalimentation," or eating too much, is a national epidemic. The American public's overeating habits are bad enough the whole year round, but then along come the holidays with the atavistic excuse for overindulgence, and the scene becomes a dietary disaster area.

Revelers sometimes rationalize their holiday behavior by

quoting the philosopher who said, "What you eat and drink between Thanksgiving and New Year's isn't all that important. What really counts is what you eat and drink between New Year's and Thanksgiving." Of course, this philosopher wasn't a diabetic. Diabetes doesn't take a holiday, and a diabetic can't take a holiday from health. So what are you to do?

Now, although there are gatherings where you won't be tempted by alcohol over the holidays (for the problem of avoiding alcohol, see "Can I drink alcohol?" on page 72), there's almost nowhere you can go where you won't be tempted by food, especially sugary food. With visions of sugarplums dancing in everyone's heads and on everyone's tables, it's going to take all your ingenuity to stick to your diet or, as we prefer to think of it, your healthful eating plan.

Let's take the last first—dessert. It's not uncommon to find two kinds of pie plus fruitcake, cookies, ice cream, whipped cream, and candy being offered with nary a morsel of plain fruit in sight. But wait. There may be *some* in sight. Look at the centerpiece. It's often a lovely display of autumnal harvest fruit and nuts. Eat it. While others give in to their addiction to concentrated sweets, just sit there and nibble upon items you've plucked from the centerpiece or other household decorations. You should rhetorically ask the host or hostess, "You don't mind if I just have a bit of this, do you? Its looks so delicious I can't resist, and it's right on my diet." What can they say? It may give them a little understanding of what the diabetic diet is for future reference. You also may start a trend at the table. When others see you've had the courage to munch on the decor, they're likely to follow suit. Many people don't feel like a heavy, sweet dessert after a large holiday meal, but they don't know how to refuse. Show them how. (One warning: make sure the fruit isn't artificial before you sink your teeth in.)

If devouring the decor is beyond your powers of brazenness, or even if it isn't, a more gracious alternative is to bring your host or hostess a fruit-and-nut gift basket. You can call it a "diabetic dessert basket" and hope you'll be offered a chance to partake of it at the end of the meal.

Another way to avoid the dessert problem and yet still make the host or hostess happy is to take *one spoonful.* After all, if you've tasted the concoction, you can praise it, and that's the most important thing. It's also a way to make yourself feel less deprived.

Let's face the final reality, though. No matter how careful you are at a big holiday dinner, you're still likely to eat more than usual. But there is one survival tactic. Exercise more than usual. Do as much of the cooking and serving as you can arrange to. If you're going to someone else's house, tell the host or hostess in advance that you'd like to help pass things, clear the table, do anything that involves motion. Most people don't realize the physical effort that goes into serving a dinner. A few Thanksgivings ago June virtually singlehandedly put on a family holiday dinner, and although she ate a good bit more than her normal diet, that night she had the worst low-blood-sugar incident of her life.

After dinner is over keep the exercises going if you can. Organize a bird- or star-viewing walk, a caroling session, a tree-trimming activity, charades with lots of physical motion—anything to keep the calories burning and the blood sugar normal. The nicest part about all these activities is that they're enjoyable in themselves.

By the way, an after-dinner activity suggested by a former president of the American Diabetes Association, Dr. Donald Bell, is testing the whole family's blood sugar. Since everyone will have had an abnormally heavy meal, it will be an appropriate time to see how their bodies handled it. Because there are those genetic factors to diabetes, you may catch a relative in the beginning stages, and he or she can get an early start on controlling it before any damage has been done. It may sound a little bizarre, but it's a good idea.

What happens if I break my diet?

If you do it once, you'll probably do it again and again and again. And each time you do it and run your blood sugar up, you risk damage to the body and the development of the serious complications of diabetes—heart disease and stroke, blindness, kidney and nerve damage, and gangrene of the feet.

The classic rationalizations are "Once won't hurt," "I can get away with it," "It's Christmas," "I can't offend the hostess," "It's my birthday," and "I'll be conspicuous if I don't." Consider yourself in a worse predicament than an alcoholic. He or she has to be a total abstainer from alcohol. You have to be a semi-abstainer from food, half on and half off the wagon at all times. A very precarious perch.

There are, however, three exceptions when we think it is okay to go ahead and cheat on your diet. In fact, we heartily recommend it. These exceptions are: (1) the day you win a gold medal at the Olympics, (2) your inaugural banquet when you're elected President of the United States, and (3) your one-hundredth-birthday party.

Of course, after all this preaching we admit that accidents will happen. Sometimes, for example, you'll inadvertently eat something that will turn out to have sugar in it. When you find yourself registering a high blood sugar after such an accident, there's no need for self-flagellation and heavy mourning. Occasional *accidental* lapses won't destroy you. (In fact, torturing yourself with frets and recriminations may do more damage to you than the dietary lapse.)

And, finally, to prove that we aren't as hard-line as we usually seem, we offer for your consideration the Hog Wild variation (see For Family and Friends: "If my diabetic child goes to a birthday party or trick-or-treating on Halloween, is it all right to break the diet just this once?" on page 185). But at the same time, we want to warn you that wild hogs can easily get out of hand and break down all barriers of self-control, and to assure you that June does not practice the hog-wild variation. *Ever.*

Is it all right for diabetics to drink sugar-free and diet sodas?

These drinks are a great breakthrough for diabetics since they allow you to be part of the group without breaking your diet. As with all things, though, a bit of moderation is in order. We heard of one man who was downing over twenty cans of sugar-free soda a day. He must have sloshed when he walked, to say nothing of the excess chemicals that must have been assailing his system.

When it comes to sugar-free drinks, a bit of caution is also in order. True story: Once when June was skiing in Deer Valley, Utah, she felt very thirsty at the end of the day. The thing she wanted most was to try a glass of the locally brewed beer, Wasatch Gold. But she'd neglected to bring her testing things along to the slopes and felt she couldn't risk the carbohydrates. Therefore, like the conscientious diabetic that she is, June marched over to the soft-drink dispenser, filled a carton with sugar-free cola, and drank it all down.

When she got back to the lodge she tested her blood sugar. It was 220! She couldn't figure it out. She'd been exercising heavily all day and had eaten and drunk only the right things. Why the high blood sugar? Our conclusion was that it had to be the cola. The person who had filled the dispenser must have used the wrong cola mix, either mistakenly or because they were out of the sugar-free variety.

We thought this was an isolated occurrence until we were talking with the former president of the American Association of Diabetes Educators, Kansas City diabetologist William Quick. He said that he and some patients and colleagues had conducted an experiment in fast-food chains in Kansas City and in Harrisburg, Pennsylvania. They tested the allegedly sugar-free drinks and discovered that one-third of them actually contained sugar.

Pat Ockel and Orchid Fickle of the SugarFree Center in Del Mar, California, corroborate Dr. Quick's findings. Pat reports that in their tests they've found lots of "sugar-free" drinks that contain sugar.

As far as we know, soft drinks in cans are safe since their quality control is a little tighter than in mix-it-yourself establishments.

You also have to train family members and friends to watch what they're buying—and pouring. After twenty years of unmitigated alertness in sugar-free-drink dispensing, Barbara absentmindedly bought a bottle of Schweppes tonic water that wasn't. For two evenings June drank it, wondering why her blood sugar was suddenly out of control every night. ("Am I coming down with something?") When she discovered the error, she was relieved to find that her diabetes hadn't become unpredictable. She was irritated with Barbara for her faulty purchase—but more irritated with herself for not taking the responsibility to always look for herself.

And a final warning on sugar-free sodas for Type I diabetics: just when you get everyone thoroughly trained to give you sugar-free drinks and nothing but sugar-free drinks, you'll probably have an insulin reaction and ask for someone to bring you a Coke *quick* and they'll dutifully grab a sugar-free one, which will do about as much good for raising your blood sugar as a cup of air. (That's another reason for always using glucose tablets for hypoglycemia: they don't make sugar-free glucose tablets.)

Why am I supposed to read the label on all food products I buy? Aren't all brands more or less alike?

Brands are not only *not* alike, they are very different. Only by reading the fine print on the label can you know, for instance, whether a certain can of grapefruit juice contains sugar. Some brands do and some don't, and it's important for you to choose a brand that is unsweetened.

It's amazing how many food products have sugar thrown in. Fruits in heavy syrup are typical. You have to really search to find the few fruits, frozen or canned, that are unsweetened. Cans of vegetables often contain sugar, as do canned meats, bottled salad dressings, frozen dinners, and endless other convenience foods. Even *salt* contains sugar—read the label if you doubt us.

There's also a confusion about many diet products. You have to realize that the term *artificially sweetened* does not necessarily mean without sugar. Drinks sweetened with saccharine often contain some sugar to counteract saccharine's bitter taste. On low-cal foods, watch for the words *sugarless* and *sugar free.* But even that's not a guarantee of safety. By law only sucrose counts as sugar, so you'll have to watch for the many chemical terms used to specify different kinds of sugars: glucose, fructose, dextrose, sucrose maltose, lactose, dextrin, and sorbitol—just to name a few (see Reference Section: How Sweet It Is, for a complete list).

The nutrition label required on food is also very helpful to diabetics. To refresh your memory, it tells the serving size, number of calories, and grams of protein, carbohydrate, and fat. This information is important to you because it can help you measure your food and fit it into your diet.

Incidentally, ingredient lists on labels are arranged according to the weight of each ingredient in descending order. The heaviest is listed first; the lightest, last. The lightest ingredients are usually those unintelligible chemical additives for which American food processors have become famous.

Can I drink alcohol?

Here you have one of the great diabetes controversies. Many doctors say absolutely no to alcohol. Not a drop. Others say it's all right in moderation. June has a joke that has a grain of truth in it. Question: "What did you do when your doctor said you couldn't drink?" Answer: "I changed doctors." There is some validity in changing doctors if you insist on drinking and he or she insists that you don't. There is no point in going to a doctor if you intend to defy instructions or, even worse, sneak off and do something forbidden.

Actually, an excellent case can be made for a diabetic not to drink at all. Even alcoholic beverages that don't contain carbohydrate, such as gin, vodka, bourbon, scotch, and dry wines, do contain calories. If you have a weight problem, the additional calories of the drink will augment this problem. If you say, "Okay, I'll figure the calories of the drink in my diet and cut out something else," you will lose the food value of that something else you cut out and your body will be deprived of the nutrition it needs.

Then, too, drinking can get you in deep trouble, especially if you're on insulin. Alcohol lowers blood sugar unless you eat while you're drinking. If you start staggering or become unconscious on the way back to your car after a visit to a bar, the police will smell the alcohol and think you're simply drunk. This is not a scenario with a happy ending.

There is the additional possibility that the alcohol may throw off your medication or alter the effect of your insulin. Some oral drugs combined with alcohol can cause nausea, sweating, and dizziness. And an out-of-control diabetic shouldn't drink a drop.

Heavy drinking can result in long-range problems for a diabetic. The journal *Diabetes Care* reported a study by David McCullogh and others of over five hundred diabetic men. The heavy drinkers in the group had a much higher incidence of painful diabetic neuropathy than the others did.

The case *for* drinking is weaker than the one against it. For many people a glass of wine is a pleasurable adjunct to a meal. It is, in fact, for some national groups as much a part of the meal as the food. One glass of wine or a single mild drink makes you feel not nearly so left out and deprived as total abstention does.

Even with your doctor's approval, however, before having a glass of anything you should do a little self-analysis of your drinking habits. We have a philosophy about diabetic drinking that we think holds true. There are two situations where a diabetic should *not* drink: The first is if alcohol means nothing to you, and the second is if alcohol means everything to you.

Whatever you drink has to be figured into your meal plan and the calories counted. Alcoholic drinks are usually calculated as fat exchanges, although you can also substitute them for bread exchanges. Naturally, you can't mix liquor with orange juice or tomato juice without counting those exchanges also. And you have to avoid such mixers as ginger ale, tonic, and other sweetened soft drinks.

The alcoholic drinks that don't contain sugar or carbohydrates are dry white wines (including champagne), dry red and rosé wines, white vermouth, whiskey, gin, vodka, scotch, rum, brandy, and tequila. A four-ounce glass of wine is about 80 calories; a four-ounce glass of vermouth is about 140 calories. The hard liquors are calculated according to their proof. The higher the proof, the more calories. As an example, eighty-six-proof alcohol is 71 calories an ounce; one hundred-proof alcohol is 83 calories an ounce. Beer is 156 calories per twelve-ounce bottle, but it also contains about the same amount of carbohydrate as a bread exchange (thirteen grams). Light beer is only 96 calories on the average and contains the equivalent of one-half bread exchange in carbohydrate. Liqueurs and cordials have to be avoided entirely as they contain sugar—sometimes as much as 50 percent sugar. Appetizer and dessert wines, like sweet sherry, port, and muscatel, are also too sweet for diabetics (see Reference Section: Carbohydrate and Calorie Values of Alcoholic Beverages).

The general recommendation is to limit alcoholic beverages to 6 percent of your daily caloric allotment. For instance, if you're on a 1,500-calorie-a-day diet, you could have one four-ounce glass of wine (80 calories) or one generous ounce of eighty-six-proof liquor (71 calories) in soda or a sugar-free mixer. You could also have it in orange juice, if you counted that as one of your fruit exchanges. If you are on a 3,000-calorie-a-day diet, you could drink twice that much (but you wouldn't *have* to, of course).

Another solution is to limit your drinking to the non-alcoholic wines and beers now available. Ariel Vineyards of California produces award-winning alcohol-free wines that have less than half the calories of wines with alcohol. Zuri of Germany has a nonalcoholic Rhine wine that contains only 130 calories per bottle. Many alcohol-free beers are now on the market in different parts of the country.

Is caffeine bad for diabetics?

By reputation, caffeine has deleterious effects on your health. It has been accused of raising blood pressure, increasing blood fats, making the heart beat faster, causing nervousness and insomnia, perhaps increasing the chance for ulcers and breast cysts, and—especially troublesome for diabetics—raising blood sugar. But shucks, a diabetic has to give up so many things, and here you have a cup of coffee (or tea) that has no calories or carbohydrates or fats and is therefore "free" in the diabetic sense of the word, a drink that Melvin Konner, M.D., writing in the *New York Times,* described as a relatively safe mood elevator. Do you have to give that up, too? Maybe not.

Recent studies indicate that for most people (even those with heart problems) caffeine causes no problem if you restrict your intake to three cups of coffee a day or less. June, who adores coffee, quickly figured out that if you drank coffee that was half decaf and half regular you could have six cups, so she started blending her own and is having enough satisfaction and oral gratification that she's not feeling the least bit deprived. If you are caffeine-sensitive or a pregnant woman or a child or have medical problems that contraindicate the use of caffeine, a better policy is to get your satisfaction from decaf drinks. Caffeine is found in many places and forms. To help you keep track of your intake, here are a few figures:

Source	Milligrams of Caffeine
Coffee (6 oz.)	110–150
Tea (6 oz.)	20–46
Diet Coke (12 oz.)	45.6
Diet Pepsi (12 oz.)	45.6
Hot cocoa (6 oz.)	2–8
Sweet dark chocolate (1 oz.)	5–35
No-Doz (1 tablet)	100
Excedrin (1 tablet)	65

What about health foods for diabetics?

If you mean home-baked bread, yogurt, soybeans, sunflower seeds, wheat germ, alfalfa sprouts, and all that, great! The more different foods you eat, the better. Just make certain that you know the calorie, protein, fat, and carbohydrate content (or exchange equivalent) of whatever you eat and limit your portions so that you stay within your diet.

June adores many health foods but finds she has to select them carefully, because many of these foods are laced with concentrated sweets—honey, coconut, dried fruits, brown sugar—and many of them are overpotent in fat and calories. For instance, one-half cup of sunflower seeds contains 280 calories and twenty-six grams of fat.

Most health breads are also heavier than ordinary bread. One slice will often equal almost two bread exchanges instead of one. You can check this out by weighing a slice. Bread is usually

50 percent carbohydrate, so a slice weighing sixty grams contains thirty grams of carbohydrate, or two bread exchanges.

DIABETES AND YOUR HEALTH

What should I expect from my doctor?

Maybe we should start off with a modification of the question "What should I expect from my doctor when first diagnosed?" This is a crucial time for you. We hope you received the examination, treatment, and care you needed and deserved at that time.

In order to give you an idea of what a first visit should involve, we consulted endocrinologist Dr. Michael Bush, director of the Diabetes Outpatient Training and Education Center at the Cedars-Sinai Medical Center in Los Angeles. He supplied a detailed account of what an ideal physical examination should be. (See Reference Section: Doctor's Initial Evaluation.)

After your first visit, you'll need to follow your doctor's recommendations for how often he or she wants to see you. It might be as frequently as three or four times a month at first. Once you get over your initial learning period and the doctor feels you're ready to be more independent, your visits may be cut down to once every three months, especially if he or she wants to order laboratory tests, such as a hemoglobin A_1C test. At each visit the doctor needs to check your testing records and go over your self-care with you to see where improvements and changes should be made. This is also your chance to ask any questions you've come up with since your last office visit.

Your doctor should also be available by telephone (or have a colleague who is available) at all times in case any serious diabetes-related emergency develops and you need help. The doctor should be willing to answer occasional questions by phone when you're having trouble handling some diabetes problem.

All this is just standard care, however. The more important

expectations you should have deal with your doctor's attitude and your interaction with him or her.

First and foremost, you should expect your doctor to treat you as an individual, not just a textbook diabetes case. You are a person with definite needs and interests and likes and dislikes, and they can and should be incorporated into your treatment. There are many different ways of handling diabetes—different diets, different exercise plans, different insulin-injection schedules that can make diabetes come at least halfway toward adjusting to your lifestyle.

In order for the doctor to make these variations on the basic theme of diabetes care, she or he is going to have to spend a little time finding out about you and your way of living, working, and playing. In other words, your doctor is going to have to talk to you. No, make that talk *with* you. There should be an interchange of ideas, not a lecture. The doctor should regard you as a colleague in your diabetes care and never convey the idea that you are incapable of understanding your condition and treatment. In fact, as Dr. Donnell B. Etzwiler says: "Diabetic patients provide 99 percent of their own care." So as your own physician you'd *better* be capable of understanding your condition and its treatment.

Your doctor, therefore, should give you a full explanation of all the laboratory tests you have. Rather than telling you your blood sugar is "normal" or "a little high, but still okay," he or she should tell you the exact figures. You should also know exactly where you stand with cholesterol, triglycerides, blood pressure—everything that affects your health and that you can make better or worse by your own behavior.

Now, although there are a lot of things that your doctor has to discuss with you, we don't want to lead you to expect that the doctor should have long, leisurely conversations with you, going over every facet of your physiological and psychological makeup. A doctor's time is too valuable to squander in great chunks. You are not the only patient, and others have their needs, too.

And speaking of time, *your* time has some value, too. You deserve a doctor who doesn't overbook and keep patients crouching in the waiting room for hours, building up stresses that are very bad for diabetes control.

This is not to say you should *never* have to wait. There are emergencies that a doctor must handle, and they can throw the schedule off, but if there is an emergency every time you have an appointment, you have cause for suspicion. We wouldn't carry on about waiting time to this extent except that since a diabetic goes to the doctor regularly every two or three months *forever,* that waiting-room time can really add up.

Since most doctors frankly admit that they lack a background in nutrition—one doctor told us he had had only a one-hour lecture on it during his entire time at medical school— you should expect your doctor to be able to refer you to a good dietitian to help you plan the complexities and personal variations of your diet. He or she shouldn't just throw a one-page diet list at you and send you on your way.

It is also extemely helpful if the office has a diabetes nurse specialist (a C.D.E.—certified diabetes educator) who can help you develop a good technique with injections, blood-sugar testing, diet, and problems of daily living. Again, these are specifics that the doctor doesn't have the time to help you with.

You should expect your doctor to keep up with the latest developments in the field of diabetes and be willing to incorporate them into your treatment.

Finally—and this may be asking too much—we personally feel that your doctor and other involved health professionals should also provide a good example. It's rather difficult for you to take good health advice from a flabby chain-smoker who is obviously ignoring all such counsel.

From all these "shoulds," you can see that it helps a great deal if your doctor is a diabetologist or an internist who specializes in diabetes.

How do I find a doctor who specializes in diabetes?

Doctors specializing in diabetes are usually listed under endocrinology and metabolism in the yellow pages. But rather than just sticking a pin in the telephone directory, you may prefer to call your local diabetes association and ask for the names of diabetologists who are closest to your home (and closeness *is* important). If your town has no local association, call your state affiliate of the American Diabetes Association and ask for a recommendation.

If you still have no luck, call your local hospital and ask who on their staff handles most of the diabetes cases.

Another good thing to do is go to your public library and check the *Directory of Medical Specialists.* This way you can find out the doctor's training, what hospitals he or she has worked in, age, and special experience. (This book is a little tricky to use. You may need to ask the librarian for help.)

We realize, however, that in some small towns there simply isn't a diabetologist. In that case, find (or keep) a doctor with whom you feel you can have a good relationship. Look for one who is willing to explore solutions to problems you present. Be sure she or he is willing to investigate new developments in diabetes that you may learn about in your reading or from discussions at meetings and seminars.

Incidentally, if you have a beloved family doctor, there's no reason to desert him or her for a diabetologist. You can keep the beloved one as your general physician and go to your diabetologist for special diabetes care.

When your diabetes is in its early stages or if you start developing problems at any time, you may want to go to one of the major diabetes clinics in the country where you stay a week or so and are given examinations and lab tests. You attend classes and learn what you need to do to get your diabetes under good control.

After all this talk about what your doctor should do for you, we mustn't forget your responsibilities to your doctor and what your doctor should expect from you.

What should my doctor expect from me?

Number one is honesty. Always tell the doctor the truth about what you're doing (or not doing) in your diabetes care. Report the true results of your blood-sugar tests. (One young woman told us she faked the results of the tests because she didn't want the doctor to be disappointed.) The doctor can't get you on the right track if he or she doesn't know that you're on the wrong one. Never try to fake the doctor out by behaving like a model diabetic for the few days just before you're scheduled for an examination and being very casual (sloppy) about your self-care the rest of the time.

You also owe your doctor cooperation. If you can't or won't follow the advice you're given, you should find another doctor whose advice you can and will accept.

Your doctor should also be able to expect you to take good care of yourself—not just your diabetes, but your *whole self.* Too many of us think we can neglect our health or even actively destroy it and then go to the doctor and say, "I'm sick. Make me well." Then if the doctor can't rectify the damage we've done, we get angry.

Don't take advantage of your doctor. If you phone constantly to discuss every little problem or try to monopolize his or her time in the office, using the doctor as a father or mother confessor, you're actually taking advantage of other patients whose time you're usurping.

It's ironic, but once you've found a doctor who is willing to listen, you have to be responsible enough to restrain yourself and stick to the facts of your diabetes problem. True, your personal problems *are* a part of the total picture of your diabetes, but a mention of their existence is enough. A diabetologist is not a psychiatrist and cannot be expected to straighten out your marriage, assuage your guilt feelings, release your inhibitions, or do whatever else is required to give you psychic peace.

If your life problems weigh unbearably upon you and you feel they are significantly detrimental to your diabetes control, ask your doctor to recommend a therapist to help you with them.

How much should I weigh?

A better question would be, What percentage of my body weight should be fat? The old height-weight-age tables are no longer considered good guides. Rather, correctness of weight should be determined by measuring the proportion of body fat and lean tissue. Simply weighing yourself is deceptive because muscle weighs more than fat, and it's the proportion of muscle to fat that counts from a health standpoint. In fact, you can be thin and still carry more fat than is healthy. When we sponsored a health-fair day at the SugarFree Center in Van Nuys, our thinnest employee—you can almost see through her—turned out to be too fat, and she was advised to lose some fat and build up more muscle. In fact, June, the only diabetic member of our Van Nuys staff at the time, was the only one who passed the test with flying colors. (It pays to be a well-disciplined diabetic.)

The recommended proportion of body fat is different for men and women. Men should be between 6 and 23 percent fat and women between 9 and 30 percent, depending on age. Men who are 25 percent fat and women who are 35 percent fat are classified as obese. There is some controversy about these recommended figures, because this is a new concept, but since you already have diabetes as a risk factor it would seem wisest to play it safe and go for the lower end of the scale if at all possible (see Table 3).

In the first edition of this book we recommended a simple pinch test to see if you were too fat. You pinch up your flesh just below your ribs at your waistline. Pressing the flesh between your thumb and forefinger, you should find a thickness of between

Age Group

Male	19-24	25-29	30-34	35-39	40-44	45-49	50-59	60+
Minimum (%)	6	6	6	6	6	6	6	6
Maximum (%)	14.8	16.5	18.0	19.4	20.5	21.5	22.7	23.5
Females								
Minimum (%)	9	9	9	9	9	9	9	9
Maximum (%)	21.9	22.4	22.7	23.7	25.4	27.2	30.0	30.8

TABLE 3. Recommended percent body fat. Although there is no established "standard" for recommended percent body fat, this table is based on the consensus of many experts in the health field. (Copyright 1987, Futrex, Inc. Reprinted by permission)

one-half and one inch. If the pinch test reveals more flesh than that, you're too fat.

A more precise way, one that will predict the exact percentage of fat, is a caliper test. This is done by taking pinches with a caliper at the midriff, on the chest, just below the shoulder, and on the front of the thigh. These results are averaged, and a table gives the corresponding fat percentage. The caliper test must be taken in a doctor's office or at a fitness center.

At the SugarFree Centers we have a Futrex-5000 Fitness and Body Composition Analyzer. This machine uses near-infrared interactance (principle: a certain wavelength is absorbed by fat but not by lean tissue) to give exact percentages of body fat. The test costs about eight dollars, and you receive not only the fat-lean analysis but a recommended body weight.

The most accurate body-composition test is naturally the most awkward and expensive. For this, you need to be weighed underwater using a hydrodensitomer. Since fat floats and muscle sinks, the heavier your are underwater, the better. (It's the opposite of the situation on land.)

It seems to us that every diabetic should seek out a place to have one of these tests and find out his or her body composition. The tests are generally available at university medical centers,

weight-loss clinics, health clubs, fitness centers, and some doctors' offices and sports-medicine centers. Incidentally, if you are
overweight according to weight charts you could find out the
happy news that your weightiness is mostly due to muscle and
therefore not risky at all. In fact, researchers did a study that
proved that overweight lean men have the same low risk of developing heart disease as normal-weight lean men. Only overweight
fat men are at greater risk.

Do I have to worry about cholesterol?

Everyone these days is either worrying about cholesterol or worrying about whether they should be worrying about it. Still cholesterol is something you should take seriously, especially if you
have diabetes. Diabetics are more likely to have higher levels of
cholesterol and blood fats (triglycerides). It may be that high
blood sugar causes elevation of LDLs (low-density lipoproteins,
or "bad" cholesterol) and lowering of HDLs (high-density lipoproteins, or "good" cholesterol). HDLs are thought to remove
cholesterol from the arteries, while LDLs lead to fatty deposits
that clog the arteries and cause heart attacks.

Thus the American Diabetes Association's *Exchange Lists
for Meal Planning* emphasizes eating vegetable fats (known as
unsaturated fats). Vegetable fats do not contain dietary cholesterol; only animal fats do. The very best of the vegetable fats
are the monounsaturated ones—avocado, canola, olive and peanut oils. Current recommendations are to eat no more than three
hundred milligrams of cholesterol a day. A book in which you
can check out the cholesterol content of different foods is Barbara Kraus's *Cholesterol Counter* (see Recommended Reading).

The newest statistics from the U.S. Center for Disease Control estimates that 60 million U.S. adults aged twenty to seventy-
four have cholesterol levels high enough to require medical
intervention. Two-thirds of these people could correct their
cholesterol levels simply by making dietary changes. The Ameri-

can Diabetes Association's recommended diet of 30 percent fat (10 percent of which may come from animal or saturated fat) is the ideal diet to keep cholesterol levels in check. Which is yet another reason being a diabetic puts you in the know about keeping healthy.

And what should your cholesterol level be? The consensus is that it should be under 200 milligrams of cholesterol per deciliter of blood; 240 is considered borderline high risk. It stands to reason that all diabetics should have regular cholesterol tests to make sure they stay under 200. Since there are now quick, inexpensive cholesterol tests using strips similar to blood-sugar-test strips, it's very simple to watch your levels. A better approach is to have your doctor take a blood sample before you have breakfast and check out your HDL and LDL levels as well as your total cholesterol. The ideal HDL level is over 50; ideal LDL is 130 or less. If you have enough HDLs you may not be at risk.

As you've probably read in newspapers and magazines, oat bran is a potent reducer of blood cholesterol. Eating oat-bran cereal or oatmeal is the best way to take advantage of oat bran's cholesterol-lowering properties. There are also supplements such as Metamucil (be sure to buy the sugar-free variety) and Fiber Excel; three daily doses of either of these can lower blood cholesterol as much as 15 percent.

Do I have to exercise?

A better question would be, Isn't it terrific that such an enjoyable activity as exercise is a basic part of diabetes therapy? The answer to both questions is yes.

Although exercise is often a neglected area in diabetes care, getting the right amount of exercise is just as important as following a good eating plan—if not more important.

We've heard it said that if you had to make a choice between eating junk food and exercising or eating a perfectly health diet and being immobile, you'd be healthier eating the junk food and exercising. Of course, a diabetic doesn't have to make that choice—in fact, can't make it. You need both exercise and good food for optimum health and blood-sugar control.

Exercise is almost a magic formula for diabetics. If you're too thin—usually the lean, insulin-dependent types—it will help you gain needed pounds by causing you to utilize your food better. Since it acts like an "invisible insulin," it helps get glucose into the cells, so less is wasted by being spilled into the urine.

If you're overweight, exercise will help you lose weight— and keep it off. Contrary to the myth, exercise does *not* increase your appetite. In fact, it suppresses it by regulating your *appestat*, the brain center that controls the appetite, and redirecting the blood flow away from the digestive tract. As a result, you'll be able to eat more because of the calories you burn, and yet you'll feel like eating less. This combination will deliver you from that complaint of so many diabetics: "I'm always hungry."

Exercise also makes weight loss easier because it revs up your metabolism, with the result that you burn more calories even when you're sitting still or sleeping. This principle is explained in Covert Bailey's well-known book *Fit or Fat?*

Besides helping overweight Type II diabetics lose weight, exercise lowers blood sugar by actually increasing the number of insulin receptors—those cell "locks" that the key of insulin is inserted into.

Exercise helps all diabetics improve circulation and lower blood fats (cholesterol and triglycerides) and therefore helps ward off the heart and blood-vessel problems to which diabetics are subject.

The benefits of exercise are not limited to physical improvements. Exercise lessens stress and is a great mood elevator. Perhaps you've heard of those brain chemicals called endorphins. Endorphins are known as the morphine within and are released when you exercise. They give you a natural high such as runners experience after about a half hour. This kind of morphine is a drug worth getting hooked on.

The only tragedy associated with exercise is that of people who have physical problems that prevent them from doing it. Diabetics who have proliferative retinopathy are warned that exercise may aggravate the problem. People with heart disease should also be aware of exercise cautions and check with their doctor before embarking on a program. And anyone with impaired circulation to the legs and feet should find out what precautions to take. Dr. Peter Lodewick, chief of the diabetes section of the Department of Internal Medicine at Zurbrugg Memorial Hospital in Riverside, New Jersey, says that such people should be particularly wary of getting blisters.

On a more encouraging note, we'd like to add that diabetes is no detriment to becoming an outstanding athlete. Some good examples are the tennis star Bill Talbert, the hockey player Bobby Clark, and, in baseball, Jackie Robinson, Ron Santo, Bill Gullickson, and Catfish Hunter.

What kind of exercise should I do?

What kind of exercise do you like? Exercise should be fun. That's the only way to be sure you'll keep doing it. As a diabetic you have enough chores in your life without turning exercise into another one.

If you want to rate exercises, though, the ones that are best for you are the aerobic or endurance kind: brisk walking, jogging, running, swimming, cross-country skiing, biking (either on the real thing or, in bad weather, on an exercycle), rowing, jumping rope. Dancing is also a wonderful endurance exercise. There are now lots of aerobics classes designed especially to build up your cardiovascular system and endurance. Several television shows can lead you through a regular aerobic session, and you can buy videotapes to do the same.

But really, as we said, exercise is play and should be fun. Try to acquire a skill you enjoy, like tennis or bowling or golf, even if it isn't an endurance sport. We find that if you get really involved in a nonendurance sport, you tend to do some endurance exercising in order to—what else?—increase your endurance for the sport you love.

Yoga is also a wonderful exercise to keep you supple, and it's something that can be done at any age.

Strengthening exercises such as weight lifting and calisthenics are okay if you like them, but they do not do the same things for general health and diabetes as endurance training.

A good exercise program for a diabetic is much the same as a good program for anyone. You should have a minimum of three sessions a week of twenty to thirty minutes. (Type II's note: you do not start burning fat until you've exercised for twenty minutes.) Don't let more than two days elapse between workouts. It's better to exercise five times a week, and to our minds exercising every day is the best, unless your body tells you not to.

Sessions should be long enough to include a warm-up and cool-down phase. Your intensity goal should be to get your heart rate to between 70 and 85 percent of its maximum capacity. To figure your training pulse range, subtract your age from 220, then multiply the result by 70 percent. The 70 percent level is sufficient to promote fitness. The 85 percent level is an upper limit, which you can sustain if you want a more intense workout. Try to maintain that rate for twenty minutes during your exercise session. (See Reference Section: Target Heart Rates.)

Before you begin an exercise program—and this is critical if you're out of shape—you should consult your physician and possibly have an exercise stress test. Your doctor may want to prescribe your heart target zone. And there is one instance in which exercise is more harmful than beneficial for diabetics. If your blood sugar is 250 or over, exercise will simply run it higher and you may produce ketones.

The best time to exercise is after meals. This way, if you take insulin or oral drugs, you're less likely to get hypoglycemic. In fact, testing before, during, and after exercise is not a bad idea until you learn your blood-sugar pattern. You may need to lower your insulin or oral drug dosage or eat extra carbohydrate. Exercise has an effect on blood sugar for twenty-four hours. So watch for hypoglycemia (low blood sugar) the day after the exercise if you've done something special like a long hike or a day of skiing.

Type I's should not inject insulin into the parts of the body that will be most used during exercise. For instance, don't inject into your legs or the arm you'll use if you're going to play tennis. The insulin would be absorbed much faster than usual if you did.

Incidentally, don't let age stop you. Even if you have health problems in addition to diabetes, there is always some form of exercise you can practice. Almost everyone can at least start walking on a schedule and then increase distance and speed until it becomes an endurance exercise.

As well as getting into a regular exercise program and sports, it's important to bring more exercise into your daily life simply by becoming a more physically active person. Get up out of your chair and move whenever possible. Climb stairs rather than taking the elevator. Park your car in the farthest corner of the parking lot and walk to the store. (Since everybody else is always trying to get as close as possible, you'll get the dividend of not having your car dinged up by the other people opening their doors on it.)

Is joining a gym a good way to get exercise?

It can be if you really go and go regularly. If you are gregarious and like to work out in the company of others, a gym may be just the motivation you need. It's a good way to get acquainted with people who have the same interest in fitness that you do. You can inspire one another—and chide one another when you don't show up. Be sure to join a gym that's not too far from your home, though, or you'll wind up spending most of your exercise time on transportation or decide not to go at all.

Belonging to a gym also has the advantage of providing

someone to watch over you when you exercise. It is important to tell people there that you're a diabetic and to explain what the symptoms of hypoglycemia are so they can spot them in the event you develop low blood sugar from exercise.

We heard peripatetic radio guru Bruce Williams say on one of his shows that when he belonged to a gym and got home from a trip, it was often too late to go to the gym or he was too tired to drive there, so he got himself a Schwinn Airdyne—an exercycle that exercises your arms as well as your legs. He said that when he got home "that darn thing was always there waiting for me and I had no excuses not to exercise." Purchasing your own exercise equipment and having it right at home might be a viable alternative for you. You could buy a new piece of equipment every year at about the cost of joining a gym. If there are others in your household who could use the equipment, it makes it an even better deal. Don't worry if you don't have a place to put it. Exercise equipment is getting more compact and portable all the time. June has an Airdyne in the garage. We have a friend who keeps her rowing machine behind the sofa in the living room. Barbara has a treadmill, a rebounder, and a rowing machine in her bedroom. This doesn't leave much space for anything else, and it doesn't enhance the decor, but health is more important than decor any day.

Walking is, of course, one of the best exercises of all, and it takes no equipment. It does have a few drawbacks, though: you can't do it in all weather, and in big cities the streets and parks are getting acutely hazardous, especially for women alone. For these reasons mall-walking is becoming a popular alternative.

So analyze yourself and choose whatever would be most likely to keep you exercising regularly. Then just do it. (P.S.: *Do it now.*)

What should I do if I'm always too tired to exercise?

To some extent, that depends on what you did to get tired. If you're weary from your job as steeplejack or longshoreman, or if you're a housewife who's cleaned the whole house or galloped after a four-year-old all day, you've already had a great deal of exercise. Getting more is not that critical for you.

On the other hand, if you're tired from a long day of sedentary office tensions or sitting in the car, you need exercise for more reasons than diabetic ones, and you should clamp your jaw and force yourself, at least initially. Just as the appetite comes with the eating, the energy and enthusiasm for exercise come with the exercising. Often the fatigue you feel at the end of the day comes from a *lack* of physical activity rather than from too much of it.

If you find yourself too tired to exercise and it's not a true physical tiredness, you may go to bed and find yourself too keyed up and tense to sleep. The next day you've got a lack-of-sleep tiredness going. Vicious cycle. But if you get out there and move those bones around, blessed sleep will descend upon you as soon as you hit the pillow. You'll sleep the sleep of the physically tired and virtuous. And you can hardly sleep a better sleep than that.

Will vitamins and minerals help my diabetes?

This question is as controversial as the question of whether vitamin and mineral pills do anybody any good. There are doctors who claim that the only thing these supplements do for most people is give them expensive urine. There are doctors who have a go-ahead-and-take-them-if-you-like attitude. And there are doctors who counsel their patients to take vitamin and mineral supplements to insure that they aren't missing anything vital in their diet.

In theory, if you are eating the healthy, balanced, and varied diet you're supposed to, you're getting your vitamins in the best way possible—from the food you eat. However, since in diabetic diets calories are often limited, taking one standard multiple vitamin a day as a safety net seems like a sound idea. Women, of course, may need to take extra iron and calcium in certain cases, but usually your physician is aware of this and prescribes the proper type and dose.

Two minerals that are often touted as helping diabetics by improving insulin usage are zinc and chromium. So far, though, we have found no studies that give any conclusive results on these two minerals for diabetics. Therefore, we favor waiting for some definite evidence of their benefits before loading up on these supplements.

One particular need for older diabetics who take diuretics is emphasized by Dr. Stephen Podolsky. He points out that these drugs can cause potassium depletion, and this, in turn, can cause your blood sugar to rise. He considers potassium depletion to be a major reason for non-insulin-dependent diabetics to be out of control. In this case, your physician might recommend a potassium supplement.

And finally, we're glad you asked "Will vitamins and minerals *help* my diabetes?" and not "Will vitamins and minerals *cure* my diabetes?" We, too, have read, in books of vitamin lore, fables of how diabetics were able to give up insulin injections entirely after loading up on vitamin supplements and health foods. Don't give yourself false hope. If you have surplus money, it's better to give it to research for a real cure for diabetes than to the vitamin industry for a false one.

What kind of eye problems can diabetes cause?

Blurred vision is one of the symptoms of long-term, out-of-control diabetes. After the diabetes is diagnosed and brought under control, vision usually returns to normal.

Because of the visual changes that can take place with changes in blood sugar, June's ophthalmologist always insists that she have normal blood sugar when she comes in to have her eyes checked to see if she needs new glasses.

When a diabetic suddenly has blurred vision or other

strange visual happenings (June sometimes reports seeing a large spot of light in her field of vision), this can indicate low blood sugar. These changes in vision can be disturbing, but they don't mean you're going blind. Blindness is always a worry for diabetics because you hear so many horrendous statistics about it. Diabetes used to be the cause of blindness in 11 percent of the legally blind people in this country, making it the third leading cause of blindness. It is still the number-one cause of new cases of blindness, but that figure may very well change in the future.

The culprit in diabetic blindness is retinopathy. This is a damaging of the blood vessels in the retina, the light-sensitive area in the back of the eye. In its later stages the delicate blood vessels of the retina may develop tiny sacs that can burst and leak blood, causing a loss of vision.

This is one of the reasons your doctor always examines your eyes so carefully: to look for changes in your blood vessels. The retina is the one place in the human body where doctors can actually see and inspect the condition of the blood vessels. Not only is weakness in the walls of the retinal blood vessels bad news in itself, but the condition of these blood vessels reflects the condition of the vessels throughout the body. You see, eyes are not just the mirrors of the soul, as the poets say, but the mirrors of the body as well.

Retinopathy is another item of the list of diabetic horribles that don't have to happen. Remember the study published in February 1989 in the *Journal of the American Medical Association*: it showed that no diabetic who had good control (less than 1.1 times normal blood sugar) had *any* eye damage, whereas of those who had blood sugar consistently above 1.5 times normal, 37 percent had retinopathy.

Even when retinopathy does develop, all is not lost. There has been a great deal of success in treating it with laser beams. As always, however, the best treatment is to keep your blood sugar normal and not develop the problem in the first place.

Why do they talk so much about diabetic foot care?

It's that same old vascular story. Diabetes can cause hardening and narrowing of the blood vessels. This, in turn, causes poor circulation of the blood. Since the feet are farthest away from the great blood pump, the heart, they get the worst deal. Poor blood circulation is also part of the aging process. So if you're older *and* diabetic, you've really got to watch those feet.

And we do mean *watch*, because if you also have a touch of neuropathy, you may not feel a cut, sore, blister, or ingrown toenail and let it go until it becomes infected. Infections are particularly hazardous because, combined with diminished circulation, they provide a welcome mat for gangrene (tissue destruction), which can necessitate amputation.

Here are the foot-care do's:

1. Wash your feet every day and wear clean socks.

2. Always dry well between your toes.

3. Cut your toenails after bathing, following the shape of the ends of the toes. Do not cut too short.

4. Wear well-fitting shoes.

5. Examine your feet daily for signs of infection.

6. If you develop foot problems, go to a podiatrist and tell him or her you are diabetic. In fact, we favor regular visits to a podiatrist.

Here are the foot-care don'ts:

1. Avoid elastic garters or anything tight around the legs or ankles.

2. Do not use heating pads or hot-water bottles on your feet.

3. Avoid smoking; it reduces the blood supply to the feet.

4. Never walk around barefoot.

5. Do not use corn plasters or any over-the-counter foot medications.

6. Do not cut corns or calluses.

7. Do not put your feet in water warmer than eighty-five or ninety degrees Fahrenheit.

If you need convincing to make you behave yourself in the foot department, the Loma Linda Diabetes Education Program offers the story of a man who didn't take care of his diabetes *or* his feet. As he aged and deteriorated, he lost his sight and all feeling in his feet. Well, it came to pass that one night, without knowing it, he knocked his watch off his bedside table and into his shoe and broke the crystal. He walked around on said broken watch for two weeks. Needless to say, he wound up as a guest in the Loma Linda Hospital.

If you are a middle-aged or older diabetic, you should watch for symptoms of diminished circulation: weak pulses in the feet and legs; cold, dry, pale skin on the feet and legs; lack of hair growth on the toes; and toes that turn a dusky red color when they hang down, as when you're sitting on the edge of the bed. Be sure to mention it to your doctor if you notice any of these symptoms.

It is possible to improve or maintain the circulation in your feet with a simple exercise. Lie on a bed with your feet raised above your hips. Alternate pointing your toes and heels toward the ceiling. Do this several times. Make circles with your feet, first clockwise, then counterclockwise. Sit up with your feet hanging over the edge of the bed. Repeat the same maneuvers as above. Do this exercise a couple of times a day.

When you get your feet in good shape, walking a mile or more daily in comfortable shoes (runners' training shoes are good) can be of great benefit.

We don't want to give the impression that older diabetics are the only ones who have to be careful of their feet. Although younger people generally have better circulation, they still can get into trouble, especially if their diabetes is out of control.

I know diabetics can have problems with their eyes and their feet, but what about their teeth?

Diabetics should pay particular attention to their teeth. Joseph E. Borkowski, D.D.S., former clinical professor at the Georgetown University School of Dentistry, wrote to us to suggest that we tell more about dentistry in relation to diabetes in this edition. He has a personal as well as a professional interest in this, since his wife was recently diagnosed diabetic. In his letter, Dr. Borkowski clearly brought out the dental concerns he has for people with diabetes:

In the treatment of any diseases of the mouth, it is important for the dentist to have as much knowledge as possible of the general health of the patient. It may seem a needless point, but the dentist must be told of a patient's diabetes. In my practice in the past I have had several instances where such information was not readily forthcoming, and some problems did arise. When necessary, the dentist will consult the physician relative to proposed treatment and whether the physician thinks changes in medication may be necessary or whether the patient's blood sugar is such that best postoperative results will be had for the patient.

It must be strongly emphasized that in patients whose diabetes is under good control, incisions and extractions heal at a normal rate. There is no doubt, however, that diabetes, when poorly controlled, will affect the patient's response to infection. When treating diabetics, it was my policy to use antibiotics on a prophylactic basis. This approach served the patient's situation well while doing no harm. The white blood cells in a diabetic whose blood sugar is high have an impaired ability to engulf and kill bacteria. Use of preoperative antibiotics could ease a potentially serious situation.

One area of concern in the mouth is tooth decay. With a diabetic, adherence to dietary management will ease this situation. Soft drinks, even those without sugar, should be avoided. That is because they have a pH of 2.3 to 2.6. (pH is a method of indicating the acidity or alkalinity of a substance. A reading of 7 is neutral; from 6 on down to 1 is progressively more acid; 8 to 14 is more base. It's easy to see that soft drinks are quite acid.) The tooth enamel consists of many small hexagonal rods held together by a cementing substance. The cementing substance is very susceptible to the action of acids; consequently, carbonated beverages break down the enamel at a high rate.

Swollen, inflamed, and bleeding gums may be a symptom of diabetes. Some part of the problem will be handled by getting the blood sugar under control.

Dr. Borkowski is an ardent advocate of the Water Pic for diabetics as a way of getting out the food that causes the bacteria in the mouth to grow and become infectious. He also advocates that diabetics use salt, baking soda, or epsom salts as tooth powder as another way to kill mouth bacteria. Following this regime is a good way for diabetics to avoid the periodontal problems to which they are susceptible.

All of Dr. Borkowski's advice on oral hygiene for diabetics wouldn't be available to his diabetic patients if he didn't know they were diabetic. If you keep the members of your health-care team in the dark about one of the physiological basics of your life, they can't do their best for you.

I wear dentures. Is there anything special I should do because of my diabetes?

For your answer, we turn again to our professor of dentistry, Dr. Joseph Borkowski, who says:

Diabetics who wear full dentures should clean them after each meal if possible. The very greatest percentage of patients I have encountered prefer to keep their dentures in at all times, taking them out only to clean them. One strong reason is that when dentures are left out all night there is usually a period of time in the morning when you have to get used to them all over again.

In a diabetic, the bone and tissue under the dentures may change more rapidly. More frequent visits to the dentist to examine for this are in order. Since full dentures do not work as well as natural teeth, cutting food into small pieces and cutting meat against the grain, will put less strain on the dentures and less wear and tear on the supporting bone and soft tissue.

Diabetic patients may develop kidney problems, which may influence the way dentures feel to them. A strong burning sensation may result, and the patient cannot wear the dentures for more than fifteen minutes. If this occurs, the dentures can be remade using a special plastic instead of the garden-variety acrylic.

Is it all right for diabetics to use hot tubs?

According to the U.S. Consumer Product Safety Commission, all people who have diabetes, a history of heart disease, or blood-pressure problems should check with a doctor on the advisability of using a hot tub.

They also caution that nobody should bathe in a hot tub with water that is 104 degrees Fahrenheit or higher, since water of 106 degrees Fahrenheit can be fatal even to fully healthy adults. (Barbara, who considers herself a fully healthy adult, gets rather frightening nosebleeds after sitting in Japanese baths or hot springs.)

The preceding section on foot care explains that you shouldn't put your feet in water warmer than 85 or 90 degrees Fahrenheit. Since it's a little awkward to soak in a hot tub with your feet hanging out, it looks as if tepid tubs should be the order of the day for diabetics.

I have a bad case of acne. Could this be caused by my diabetes?

Possibly. Some diabetics report that they have acne when their diabetes is out of control and that it clears up when their blood sugar is stabilized.

Then again, it's possible that your acne has nothing to do with your diabetes. Many diabetics have a tendency to figure that every physical problem from acne to Zenker's diverticulum of the esophagus is related to their diabetes. When June had chronic headaches, she at first thought they were caused by low blood sugar. It turned out they had nothing to do with diabetes.

It is true that diabetes, especially out-of-control diabetes, can cause a variety of minor and not-so-minor health problems. Still, you should try to avoid laying the blame for everything on diabetes. Not only does this make you feel more depressed and put upon, but it may also cause you to delay seeking treatment for whatever your problem really is.

Are flu shots necessary for diabetics?

They don't always work because there are often so many different strains of flu going around that you get zapped by one your shot doesn't cover. Still, we think they're a good idea. Flu can upset control of blood sugar for insulin takers, and flu shots are usually recommended for older people. Put those two groups together and you've just about covered the whole diabetic population.

Since flu shots themselves can cause rather heavy flu symptoms in susceptible beings, it's sometimes wise to take two half doses at different times. June always does this with flu shots and with shots she has to take for foreign travel as well.

Why do doctors always insist that diabetics give up smoking?

Smoking is dangerous for everyone, but doubly dangerous for diabetics. Inhaling cigarette smoke affects the blood vessels. Diabetes can affect the blood vessels. Both diabetes and smoking tend to narrow them, and narrowed arteries can cause heart disease and gangrene.

An out-of-control diabetic has 2.5 times the normal chances of getting heart disease. A smoker has 1.7 times the normal chances of dying of heart disease. Put the two together and you have over 4 times the normal risk of heart disease.

An out-of-control diabetic has 60 times the normal chances of getting gangrene of the feet. Again, smoking increases that already dismal figure.

A study done at the University Hospital in Copenhagen, Denmark, found that diabetic patients who smoked required 15 to 20 percent more insulin than nonsmokers. Their level of blood fats was also higher.

You might call smoking a kind of Virginia roulette for diabetics. So why are there diabetic smokers? That's a question we have no answer for, except that their use of nicotine is an addiction harder to kick than an addiction to heroin. So people try and fail and try and fail ad infinitum.

The best suggestion we have is to seek help. Without help, your chance of quitting (and not relapsing) is slim indeed. A government survey found that only about 10 percent of the smokers who want to quit seek help. That is thought to be the reason why so few succeed.

Where can you get help? Many hospitals now have clinics or treatment centers specializing in smoking-cessation programs. There are independent programs too, like Smokenders and Schick. Ask your doctor for advice. Just be sure the system you try addresses all the dependency problems of smoking: the physical, the psychological, and the social. As Dr. Judith Ockene, director of preventive and behavioral medicine at the University of Massachusetts Medical Center, pointed out in a *New York Times* article, "the most effective methods deal with a smoker's three-pronged dependency and recognize that quitting is a process—not a one-time event—that occurs three or four times over five to ten years."

DIABETES AND YOUR DAILY LIFE

Should I tell people I have diabetes?

In general, definitely yes. You should tell everyone you have any kind of regular, everyday contact with—your hairdresser or barber, your colleagues at work, your teachers, your coaches, your friends (even rather casual ones), and especially those with whom you play sports.

You should make it a special point to tell anyone with whom you have any kind of medical or semimedical dealings, such as your dentist or podiatrist or oculist, because that may influence their treatment of you.

There are several good reasons for letting people know you have diabetes, especially if you are insulin-dependent. In the first place, should you have an insulin reaction, a person in the know can help you out or at least will realize that whatever is happening to you may be related to your diabetes and will get you to someone who can help.

You are also much less likely to inadvertently offend people if they know you have diabetes. For example, if you get low blood sugar and suddenly turn into a grouch or hellion, they may realize it's because of your diabetes, not because of a mean streak that's part of your nature. Then, too, if you're eating at a friend's house and turn down a sugar-shot confection, the cook will know that you're not insulting his or her culinary talents but just behaving yourself and dutifully following your own diabetic diet.

Another reason for informing people about your diabetes is that you can help out other diabetics by educating nondiabetics as to what diabetes is. What diabetics need is an each-one-teach-one program in order to spread diabetes facts and wipe out some of those weird fictions that are floating around in the public mind, such as "Diabetics can't eat sugar, but they can eat all the honey they want because honey is natural."

If you do tell others about your diabetes, you're also likely to find that you are not as alone in your condition as you thought. Almost everyone you mention your diabetes to will start telling you about a diabetic cousin or grandmother—or even about their diabetic selves!

As part of your diabetes announcement program, you should certainly wear some sort of identification bracelet or medallion. This is a safeguard in case you are ever in an accident or have some sort of diabetic problem when you're away from those who know you. A particularly good identification is a Medic Alert bracelet (available from Medic Alert Foundation, Turlock, California 95381-1009, 1-800-ID ALERT). Medic Alert is well known now, and ambulance attendants, members of the ski patrol, and nurses in emergency hospitals are on the lookout for its insignia.

Now, after advocating this policy of extreme honesty, we'll hedge a bit. You don't have to be obsessed with your diabetes and immediately tell everyone you meet, "Hello-there-I'm-John-Smith-and-I'm-a-diabetic-pleased-to-meet-you," any more than you'd announce to a new acquaintance that you have gallstones or are color-blind or wear a pacemaker. As you get to know people better, your diabetes will emerge appropriately and naturally as a subject for conversation.

As for telling prospective employers and insurance agents, it's a yes-and-no situation that we'll discuss shortly.

Which is the correct thing to say: "I am a diabetic," or "I have diabetes"?

Either is correct. It's a matter of personal preference. The journal *Diabetes in the News* once ran a reader survey to see which most diabetics prefer. "I am a diabetic" won a clear victory. Most people thought it was more straightforward and more accepting of your condition.

A case can be made, however, for "I have diabetes." It sounds more as if you are giving yourself primary importance and your disease only secondary importance. You're a person who just happens to have diabetes.

Either of these phrases will make you easily understood. Don't shy away from them and use something cryptic the way June did once on a flight to Hawaii, when she was trying to get her meal from the flight attendant. "I'm on insulin," she said. "Could you serve me first?" The answer was negative. The problem, we figured out later, was that the flight attendant, who was Danish, didn't have any idea what June was talking about. In fact, she probably thought that insulin was the name of some kind of group tour of the islands and that June was just trying to get a special privilege for no good reason.

When Barbara trotted back a few minutes later and made eyeball-to-eyeball contact with the flight attendant and announced, "My friend is a di-a-bet-ic and she needs to eat. Could you serve her now?" the meal appeared a few seconds faster than immediately.

Experts have very definite ideas about correctness in the use of the words *diabetes* and *diabetic*. They don't like you to use *diabetic* as an adjective, unless what you're talking about actually has diabetes. For example, "The diabetic man had a diabetic dog" is all right, because both the man and the dog are diabetics. "The diabetic education lecture was held at the diabetic study center" is all wrong, because neither the education lecture nor the study center has diabetes. It should be "The diabetes education lecture was held at the diabetes study center."

You wouldn't say "a diabetic specialist" unless the specialist you're talking about has diabetes. If he's a specialist in diabetes, he should be called a diabetes specialist. If he's a specialist in diabetes who has diabetes, then presumably he'd be referred to as a "diabetic diabetes specialist." But maybe you think this is being linguistically nitpicky. Maybe we think so, too; since, as you may notice, we often use the word *diabetic* in the unaccepted way, and, in fact, interchange *diabetic* and *diabetes*, especially when referring to the diet.

Just to put the capper on the whole nomenclatural confusion, the British call their organization the British Diabetic Association. But they always did have trouble with the language.

Will I be able to get insurance as a diabetic?

That depends on the kind of insurance you're interested in getting.

Automobile insurance. There should be no trouble if you're in good control. (Here's yet another reason to take good care of yourself.) If they ask on the form if you're a diabetic, naturally you have to tell them. In that case, they'll probably ask you to produce a letter from your doctor saying that your diabetes is under control.

If they don't ask, we don't see any point in saying "Hey there, insurance company, I'm a diabetic. Don't you want to hassle me?" Personal experience: June's automobile insurance company has never asked; she has never told.

Life insurance. If you're in control (again with evidence required) and you take less than forty units of insulin—or don't take insulin at all—you should have no more difficulty getting life insurance than a nondiabetic.

Health insurance. If you or your spouse—or, in the case of minors, your parents—work for a company or government agency with a group plan, you'll be taken care of, diabetic or not. If you have to take out an individual policy, then, as a study reported in *Diabetes in the News* put it, "your chances are . . . mighty slim." In all likelihood you may not be able to get a policy at all or it will cost too much to even think of or there will be a huge deductible (we've heard of some as high as two thousand dollars) or they may try to exclude coverage for all diabetes-related problems. This last stipulation would be particularly ludicrous: insurance companies being how they are, they'd find a way to say your diabetes was the cause no matter what happened. Cardiovascular problem? Of course, diabetes did it! Infection? Naturally, diabetics are notoriously susceptible to infections. Run over by a truck? Sure thing! You probably had hypoglycemia and walked into its path.

The SugarFree Center currently has twelve employees eligible for health insurance. Five of these employees are diabetic. One of our employees has a diabetic daughter, so that makes six diabetics altogether. Until April 1989 we were owned by a large health corporation, so everyone got health insurance with no problem.

Then our company was divested from the corporation, and we formed another small corporation and innocently set out to find insurance coverage for our employees. After contacting thirty-four different companies, we found that we could get insurance only if all the diabetics were excluded from coverage of their "preexisting condition" for twenty-four months. Since, as you know, diabetes is an expensive disease—and two of our employees are on infusion pumps, which makes it even more expensive—to have no coverage for diabetes for twenty-four months would be a terrible hardship.

Because our employees were terminated by the old corporation, we thought that the government's COBRA plan (which allows you to get health-insurance coverage for eighteen months when you're terminated from a job) would bridge the gap. Although it would be horribly expensive, we figured that for the diabetics we could have both plans run concurrently. That way they would have a gap in their diabetes coverage for only the six months after the COBRA plan ran out and before the new insurance kicked in.

No such luck. The friendly federal government said that if a company had an insurance policy for its employees, it couldn't have a COBRA plan as well since COBRA is only for those who have no other health insurance. "But," we squeaked, "our diabetic employees *don't* have any insurance for their diabetes for twenty-four months." The reply was the government equivalent of "hard cheese."

But we shouldn't feel picked on because we're diabetic. As Henry Helfman, an insurance agent (and a diabetic), explained to us, individual health-insurance policies are a pretty rotten deal for everyone, with high prices and exclusions galore. He goes so far as to advise everyone to get into a group plan if at all possible—even if it means changing jobs. In the college library where we formerly worked, there were women who took clerical jobs mainly to get the excellent health benefits for themselves and their families. That makes a certain amount of sense. So if you have a choice between two jobs and everything else is equal, you'd be wise to select the one with the better health plan.

The only real solution, though, is some kind of state pooled-risk plan or federal universal health insurance for diabetics and others with chronic health problems. States with pooled-risk plans mandate that health-insurance companies doing business in that state contribute to a fund to make health insurance available to people considered "uninsurable." This insurance must have a maximum premium charge of no more than 125 to 150 percent of that particular state's average premium. If you live in one of the eighteen states that currently have pooled-risk plans, you're in luck. The states are Connecticut, Florida, Georgia, Illinois, Indiana, Iowa, Maine, Minnesota, Montana, Nebraska, New Mexico, North Dakota, Oregon, South Carolina, Tennessee, Texas, Washington, and Wisconsin. Check with your insurance agent on how to get onto one of these plans, or if that fails, contact your state health department.

But no matter how bad it looks at the moment, the health-insurance situation is *not* hopeless. It's rather like having diabetes. There can be a successful outcome, but only through your own dedicated efforts. If your state doesn't have pooled risk, write your state legislators about it. And while you're at it, write your congresspeople and senators asking for federal insurance coverage. Do this even if you're fortunate enough to have health-insurance coverage. Do it for your fellow diabetics and for those who have other chronic diseases. And do it for yourself. You never know. Your employment situation might change, leaving you out in the cold without the warm coat of insurance coverage.

Medicare. No discussion of health insurance would be complete without a few harsh words for Medicare. James Herndon wrote a book a few years back about the dismal state of education in the inner-city schools and how, as the students put it, things were "supposed to be" but weren't. In theory, Medicare is *supposed* to provide a lot of benefits to diabetics for their self-care. In practice, it often provides a stress-raising adventure in frustration and failure for the diabetic.

In the first place, unless you take insulin, you're totally out of luck; Medicare will provide nothing for your diabetes care. If you do take insulin, ironically, Medicare neither pays for your basic life necessities—insulin and syringes—nor does it pay for alcohol swabs, tax, or shipping charges. (And, of course, it doesn't pay for anything until the annual deductible has been met.) Even if you're insulin-dependent, it won't pay for blood-sugar-testing equipment and supplies unless your physician fills out a questionnaire indicating that you have complications and/or are usually out of control. Wise doctors always paint as bleak a picture as possible on the questionnaire. If you meet the above criteria, Medicare is *supposed* to provide 80 percent of up to $180.77 for a blood-sugar-testing meter. (Note: Medicare will pay for *no* supplies without a meter.) After the meter purchase, Medicare will currently pay 80 percent of up to $95 a month for necessary supplies. The supplies that they're *supposed* to cover include test strips, strip-splitting devices, instruments for pricking the finger, cotton balls, batteries for monitors, control and calibration fluids, calibration chips, and confidence strips to check a meter's accuracy.

The real fun begins when you file a claim on any of these

supposedly covered items. During one disastrous year when we were Medicare suppliers and had no insurance expert on the staff as we now do, Medicare sent back half the claims we filed. Sometimes they sent them back as many as six times. Usually they rejected a claim by saying we hadn't sent in a prescription or the questionnaire even though we had. Several times they turned down a claim for a meter because we hadn't stated for how long the person would be using it. (Marian, in our customer-service department, a Medicare recipient herself, wryly wrote back that we assumed Medicare realized that diabetes was a lifetime disease and we had no ability to predict the length of the life of the meter purchaser.) Our employee processing Medicare claims said she noticed that whenever the claim was over one hundred dollars, Medicare seemed to find some excuse to turn it down.

Even if Medicare ultimately paid, it was a very slow process. We later read in an *AARP News Bulletin* that this is deliberate. To slow down outgoing cash flow, the Health Care Financing Administration has asked Medicare contractors to increase the backlog of claims to be paid to Medicare beneficiaries. "The increased backlog will mean that by the end of [the year] some beneficiaries will have to wait up to twice as long before receiving reimbursement," said the article.

There are *supposed* to be a lot of improvements in Medicare coverage coming round the bend. Beginning in 1991, Medicare is *supposed* to pay 50 percent of prescription-drug costs over $600, and 80 percent by 1993. This would mean that those who take oral hypoglycemics would be covered. We asked our director of pharmacy services, Mike Voelker, if insulin and syringes might slip in under the wire, too, since they're under prescription in some states. He said we won't know until we get the final information on the plan. We've also seen reports in the newspaper of rumblings out of Washington that the proposed new Medicare coverage would be such a fiscal burden that the nation couldn't handle it and changes might have to be made.

In the meantime, when it comes to making Medicare claims, based on our experience and that of others, we offer the following advice:

1. Never assume Medicare will pay for anything, even the things they're *supposed* to. If you don't want a certain piece of equipment or supplies unless you can be certain that Medicare will pay or that it will pay fairly promptly, it would be best not to take the chance.

2. Have your doctor write the prescription for the meter simply as "blood-glucose monitor and necessary supplies for lifetime use." If he or she puts down a specific meter by name, the particular name may not be in the Medicare computer and the claim will get turned down.

3. Always keep a copy of anything you send to Medicare. In fact, keep several copies. They're likely to ask for them again and again and again.

4. Please don't shout and scream and throw things at physicians, hospitals, and other providers who are nice enough to file your Medicare claims for you. They're only trying to help, and if things get fouled up and claims don't get paid, 99 percent of the time it's Medicare's doing, not theirs.

5. Keep your sense of humor operative. You'll need it!

Will diabetes keep me from getting a job?

It didn't keep actress Mary Tyler Moore, radio and TV personality Gary Owens, hockey star Bobby Clarke, prominent physician Peter Forsham, or McDonald's restaurant tycoon Ray Kroc from getting the jobs they wanted. Why would it keep you from any career you choose? The truth is that the great majority of diabetics have the same employment opportunities and limitations as nondiabetics. So if you're qualified for a particular position, go after it positively and aggressively. Be up-front about your diabetes. If the subject comes up with an employer, point out that diabetes develops a sane lifestyle and great self-discipline. These in turn lead to superior performance on the job.

We have two examples of young men seeking their heart's choice of career—to be a doctor—in spite of being Type I diabetics. Their experiences also demonstrate the difference between then and now, between the old days of prejudice and discrimination against diabetics and the new ones of open opportunity.

Then

George L. Chappell, M.D., a psychiatrist practicing in Ventura, California, has been a diabetic for over thirty-seven years now. He knew from the age of four that he wanted to be a physician, so he actually overqualified himself during high school and college: high grades, a job, community volunteer service, everything to show he could succeed and carry a heavy workload. He applied to twenty medical schools and was rejected by all of them. One admissions officer told him: "Well, George, your qualifications are certainly way above average, but you're not going to live long enough for society to regain the investment that it makes in your education, so we won't be able to accept you." But Dr. Chappell persisted, pulling every string he could until finally the admissions officer at the University of California at Los Angeles caved in. He is still very much alive and has found the struggle well worth it, as "the emotional and professional rewards are great." He says that because of diabetes, he has a degree of empathy and personal experience that physically healthy physicians lack. Many of his patients notice his special concern and are grateful to have found such an out-of-the-ordinary therapist.

Now

Our first employee at the original SugarFree Center in Van Nuys, California, Ron Brown, joined us the summer before he planned to enter a Ph.D. program in psychology. As a diabetic himself, he had an instant rapport with all of our clients and, because of his deep reading in the field of diabetes, was invaluable in providing support and counseling.

The warm feelings that our clients felt toward Ron were obviously reciprocated. He soon knew that he wanted to devote his life to working with diabetics. Because of his talent for gourmet cooking and because he saw the difficulty most diabetics have in understanding and adjusting to the dietary changes their disease requires, he decided to work toward his R.D. degree.

After his swift and successful completion of the R.D. program at the University of California at Berkeley, he came back to work with us at the Del Mar, California, SugarFree Center and served as a dietitian at the nearby Scripps Clinic. His increased experience in diabetes at Scripps and with us heightened his interest in the field and made him realize that to do as much as he wanted to do to help other diabetics, he would have to become a physician. Therefore, on top of working both at Scripps and at the SugarFree Center, he took the additional premed courses he lacked.

Ron applied for entrance to medical school in 1986 at the age of thirty. Both his age and his diabetes could have worked against him. Neither did. He was accepted by three medical schools without a quibble and probably would have been accepted by more except that he withdrew his other applications when he was accepted at the one he really wanted, the University of California at Davis. He has now finished his first two years with flying colors, and June is looking forward to having him as her doctor in the very near future.

Not only does Ron's story show that prejudices against diabetes in the work world are crumbling, but it poses an interesting question. Would he be where he is today—getting ready to embark on a medical career—if he had not developed diabetes? As our supervising nurse-educator, Elsie Smallback, always says, "out of something bad comes something good."

Ron's story reminds us of what we read about prize-winning novelist Walker Percy. He had gone to medical school because it was the thing to do in his family. After graduation he decided to go into psychiatry and interned at Bellevue Hospital in New York. He never practiced, though, because he contracted pulmonary tuberculosis and spent three years recuperating. For much of that time he was flat on his back, reading voraciously, mostly fiction and philosophy, which ultimately led to his literary career. He calls tuberculosis "the best disease I ever had. If I hadn't had it, I might be a second-rate shrink practicing in Birmingham at best."

Some years from now, it will be interesting for you to muse awhile on how your life has changed *for the better* because of your diabetes. You may well be surprised at what you come up with.

Realistic optimists that we are, however, we do have to report a few—very few—negatives in career selection for diabetics who take insulin. You should avoid jobs where you could endanger yourself or others during insulin reactions. It wouldn't be wise for you to seek jobs that involved high-speed machinery or climbing around on skyscraper construction girders, for example. Legally, there are certain restrictions, too. The federal government does not allow diabetics on insulin to enter the armed forces, to pilot airplanes, or to drive trucks or buses in interstate commerce.

If you should run into job discrimination because of diabetes, don't hesitate to fight it. Federal regulations have made it illegal for most major employers to reject you solely because you have diabetes. You can file a complaint if you run into this situation. The law that protects you is Title V of the Rehabilitation Act passed by Congress in 1973. For details on how to file, write the American Diabetes Association (see Reference Section: Directory of Organizations).

FOR MEN: Will my diabetes cause sexual problems?

According to early statistics, between 40 and 60 percent of diabetic men are ultimately affected by impotence. (A variation on this statistical theme is that the incidence of impotence is 15 percent in diabetic men between the ages of thirty and forty and 55 percent by age fifty.) As Mark Twain said, "There are lies, damned lies, and statistics." These statistics are probably akin to the now false figures about how many diabetics go blind or have amputations and kidney failure—all computed from the period when we didn't have the therapies we now have to keep blood sugar normal.

We actually hate to even quote these impotence statistics since reading them is just the sort of thing that could cause it. One psychologist we heard at a conference recounted the story of one of his patients who wasn't aware of the existence of diabetic impotence and was getting along just fine. When he heard the discouraging word, it was instant impotence for him. So if you're not having any problems in that line and if you're keeping your blood sugar normal, forget the statistics and go on with your life—and your sex life. If you've had or are having some problems or harbingers thereof, read on.

First of all, the impotence legends reflect several factors. Sometimes when a man is an undiagnosed, out-of-control diabetic, he can develop a *temporary* impotence, which goes away when his diabetes is diagnosed and he gets his blood sugar back in the normal range. This has inflated the statistics cited above.

Second, when diabetes is first diagnosed, a man is shot with so many negative emotions—such as anxiety, depression, anger, guilt, fear of rejection, and worry over his future—that he becomes impotent for psychological reasons, not because of his diabetes.

Sometimes the problem is caused by what sex therapists William H. Masters and Virginia E. Johnson call "spectatoring." Raul C. Schiavi and Barbara Hogan, writing in *Diabetes Care,* vividly describe the situation in which a diabetic man has heard the statistics and wonders if he's going to be a victim of them: "The diabetic patient, rather than becoming involved in the sexual experience and abandoning himself into erotic sensations and feelings, may find himself constantly monitoring the state of his penis. He becomes a witness rather than a participant in the sexual experience." Not surprisingly, this "performance anxiety" often results in impotence.

Indeed, the *British Medical Journal* reported that diabetic impotence was most likely caused by psychological factors in two-thirds of the men studied and by physical factors in only one-third. On the other hand, the brochure of the Recovery of Male Potency Program at Grace Hospital in Detroit says, "Twenty years ago, most doctors thought that impotence was primarily a psychological problem. We now realize that 80 percent of impotence has a physical rather than a psychological cause." And Ginger Manley, R.N., M.S.N., writing in the *Diabetes Educator*, states, "While in the general population only about 50 percent of impotence is physical in origin, in the diabetic population physically mediated impotence approaches 90 percent." (You read your statistics and you take your choice.) In short, impotence can be a combination of physical and psychological factors.

An easy and inexpensive way for you to determine if impotence is psychological or physical has been suggested by the broadcaster-columnist Dr. Gabe Mirkin. He explains that there are two stages of sleep: rapid-eye-movement (REM) and non-rapid-eye-movement sleep. In non-rapid-eye-movement sleep, males achieve an erection. This can occur several times throughout the night, and the male wakes up the next morning without even knowing it happened.

If you are achieving erections in the night, your impotence is psychological. To check this out, Dr. Mirkin recommends taking a roll of postage stamps (the one-cent kind, for thrift's sake), tearing off the appropriate number of stamps (he suggests four), and securing them tightly to the penis before going to bed. If the stamps are torn apart in the morning, you know you're having erections.

To make sure that anxiety resulting in fitful sleep doesn't confuse the issue, it might be a good idea to try this test more than once before deciding that your impotence is physical rather than psychological.

What can I do about impotence that is mainly psychological?

We hope it will help some just to have the ressurance that it *is* mainly psychological and that when you start handling the negative emotions that engulfed you with your diagnosis of diabetes the sex problem will gradually disappear.

We know, however, that such emotions and their effects can't always be swept away with logic and Dutch-uncle conversations with yourself. You can't immediately eliminate your problem just because you've been told what's causing it. It takes time and consideration (consideration of yourself by yourself as well as consideration from your partner). If it takes too much time— and only you can decide how much is too much—you shouldn't hesitate to get some psychological help.

If your doctor isn't able to recommend a psychological counselor or sex therapist, you can contact any large university in your area. Most of these have human-sexuality programs and can give you the names of qualified sex therapists who are available for private consultation. And it is imperative that both you and your partner go to the therapist.

What can I do about impotence that is caused by physical factors?

Richard K. Bernstein, M.D., in his book *Diabetes: The GlucograF™ Method for Normalizing Blood Sugar,* suggests that if impotence in Type I diabetics is occasional and if it occurs during the first five to ten years of the disease, the "inability to become aroused or, if aroused, inability to achieve orgasm can be an early warning of hypoglycemia [low blood sugar]. . . . This early warning sign has been detected by both males and females. In fact, patients have located the blood-sugar levels at which they 'turn off.'" He continues, "It appears that both men and women tend to have two turnoff points: at one blood-sugar level they can be aroused but cannot achieve orgasm; at a lower blood-sugar level they cannot even be aroused. . . . Some patients try to prevent an unpleasant situation by measuring blood sugar when feasible prior to anticipated intercourse and promptly take fast-acting sweets if blood sugar is low."

You can also become impotent while under the influence of certain drugs. Among these are alcohol, tranquilizers, marijuana, and estrogens, so check with your doctor. In many older men, impotence may be caused by hypertension drugs, with diabetes getting the blame. When possible, these suspect drugs should be avoided or their use discontinued. Your physician may be able to suggest an alternative medication.

Most long-range, gradually occurring impotence in diabetics is due to one or a combination of three factors:

1. a decrease in the male hormone, testosterone. This is the least likely of the three. It can be treated with hormone injections.

2. an interruption of the blood flow to the penis, usually as a result of atherosclerosis (hardening of the arteries).

3. neuropathy—damage to the nerves that carry the sexual message from the brain and dilate the blood vessels. This neuropathy is usually caused by long-term poor control of blood sugar and is sometimes reversible with improved control.

Some treatments that have proved successful include injections of drugs that improve the supply of blood to the penis, the use of vacuum-constriction devices, and penile implants. The implants can be rigid, semirigid, or inflatable. Anyone seeking help with physiological impotence should consult with a urologist. There are also many hospitals now setting up impotency programs where the problem of impotence can be evaluated, the options explained, and corrective procedures instituted. These programs often include invaluable support groups.

There is also an excellent article on the subject of impotence: *Diabetes and Sexual Health* by Ginger Manley, R.N., M.S.N., which appeared in volume twelve, number four of the *Diabetes Educator*. If you can't locate it in a local medical library, you can write to the American Association of Diabetes Educators for a copy (see Reference Section). Another good source of information is Impotents Anonymous, 119 S. Ruth St., Maryville, Tennessee 37801, 615-983-6404.

It's important to remember that with impotence, as with all problems associated with diabetes, the best treatment is no treatment—that is to say, preventive maintenance that keeps the problem from developing in the first place. As Dr. Neil Baum, director of the New Orleans Impotence Foundation, says, "Men with poorly controlled diabetes have decreased sex drive as well as problems with impotence. Good control is associated with improvement in potency, libido, and sense of well-being."

FOR WOMEN: Will my diabetes cause sexual problems?

Previously it had been thought that diabetes had little or no effect on either a woman's sexual performance or satisfaction. Even now, based on what diabetic women report to their doctors, it would seem that they reach a sexual climax just as often as nondiabetic women.

Still there are rumblings from some diabetes therapists—especially female diabetes therapists—that sex problems associated with diabetes are as common among women as among men. It's just that the male sex problems have been given more attention. This is not necessarily due to sexism. It may be due to the fact that sexual response is easier to measure with men than with women. (And easier for women to fake than men.)

The majority of women's sexual problems appear to be related to poor diabetes control. A woman understandably loses interest in sex when she is excessively tired and run down from being out of control. High blood sugar and the resulting sugar in the urine increase susceptibility to vaginal infections that cause swelling, itching, burning, and pain, which are hardly conducive to enthusiasm for sexual intercourse. These infections can be treated with salves, but the only real cure is keeping your diabetes under control.

If a long-term diabetic woman develops neuropathy (damaged nerve cells)—again often as a result of poor control—it may involve the nerve fibers that stimulate the genitalia so that arousal may not occur, making intercourse painful because lubricating fluids are not released. Arthur Krosnick, M.D., writing in *Diabetes Forecast,* recommends the use of water-soluble lubricants, such as K-Y Lubricating Jelly, for this condition. He also states that "estrogen deficiency responds to vaginal creams. These creams are available by prescription and do not affect diabetes control."

Emotional factors associated with diabetes—anxiety, fear, anger, and, especially, depression—can significantly decrease a woman's desire for sex, especially since these negative emotions often result in (or are a result of) poor diabetes control.

Dr. Lois Jovanovic-Peterson, writing in *The Diabetic Woman,* neatly sums up the situation: "The best way to be sexy and enjoy sex, therefore, is to be happy, healthy, fit, and in good control of your blood-glucose levels."

She also offers this handy hint for insulin-taking diabetic women when things are going well in the sex department: "If a woman thoroughly enjoys the sexual encounter, the sheer exercise of the experience may result in a severe hypoglycemic episode. Thus, a woman needs to be prepared. She should adjust her insulin downward in anticipation of the evening, or if the evening happens to be on the spur of the moment, she should compensate by eating something afterward." *Bon appétit!*

Should I become pregnant?

We assume from this question that you have already wrestled through the basic Everywoman life decision of whether to have children and have concluded that you want to, but you worry about the effect your diabetes will have on your baby and vice versa.

The first consideration is: do you have any diabetes complications such as retinopathy (diabetic eye damage), neuropathy (nerve damage), or poor kidney function? If so, you may have to postpone the idea of becoming pregnant, because pregnancy could worsen the condition. Oddly enough, it can go both ways. In the case of retinopathy, Dr. Jovanovic-Peterson told us that "of one hundred women with retinopathy, 50 percent have no change, 25 percent get better, and 25 percent get worse with pregnancy." It is for this reason that before entering into a pregnancy you need to consult with your diabetes specialist to make sure you have a normal hemoglobin A_1C, with you gynecologist, with an ophthalmologist, and with a urologist.

If all systems are go, you can be cheered by the news that your chances of having a healthy baby are exactly the same as a nondiabetic woman's. The one great warning is to establish normal blood sugar (a normal A_1C) *before* becoming pregnant. Otherwise, you're in trouble from the start.

We must also forewarn you that a diabetic woman's pregnancy means a great intensification of self-care. Blood sugar must be monitored on a meter between five and ten times a day. Blood-sugar level must be kept between 60 and 90 before meals and less than 140 after meals during the entire term of the pregnancy. This means excessive risk of hypoglycemia for Type I's.

That's why the pregnancy is sometimes harder on the husband than the wife.

Cost is also an important factor. The major expenses are blood-sugar-testing supplies and fetal monitoring (amniocenteses, ultrasounds, fetal-echo checks, and fetal nonstress tests). Not to scare you, but the cost of fetal testing for one of our SugarFree Center employees was $3,650 in 1987.

If your main concern involves the ethics of producing a child with the possibility of diabetic heredity, that's a decision only you can make. Fortunately, the pattern of inheritance of diabetes is now much clearer, and the picture looks brighter than it did just a few years ago. Children of Type I diabetics have only a 2 to 6 percent chance of also becoming diabetic. Non-insulin-dependent diabetes is more inheritable. The children of Type II's have a 15 to 25 percent chance of becoming diabetic.

What is the best contraceptive for a diabetic woman to use?

Birth control for diabetic women is essentially the same as for nondiabetic women. The choice is up to the woman, her mate, and her gynecologist. The most commonly used method is the low-dose pill. These pills are not considered dangerous unless you have high blood pressure or retinopathy. Ordinarily they do not have an impact on your insulin doses, but in higher dosages they can change insulin requirements and thus it's best to keep in touch with your diabetes doctor and gynecologist about this.

The long-standing barrier methods are okay, also—diaphragms, condoms, and cervical sponges. For women who are certain they don't want to become pregnant in the future, sterilization (obviously) is the most reliable method.

One diabetic woman we talked to said she thinks the safest and most reliable method of contraception is a husband with a vasectomy.

And, finally, our editor, who feels we should present every

possible option in this book, offers the reminder, "There's always celibacy."

Can diabetics travel?

Anyone who knows the two of us at all will realize that we would consider that question as ridiculous as asking "Can diabetics breathe?" Travel is that much a part of our lives—and we feel it should be that much of a part of yours.

On this shrinking planet, your job may require you to travel all over the country or even all over dozens of other countries. Never let your diabetes stop you. If you keep yourself under good control and plan ahead, you'll make business trips with as much ease and success as the nondiabetic next person. As a matter of fact, because of your good health habits, you may well be brighter and more alert and ready for the work than nondiabetics, who may feel a little headachy from airline cocktails or drowsy from carousing.

Terrence Mason, a trainer for the Grantmanship Center in Los Angeles, spends an estimated 60 to 70 percent of his time traveling all over the world. In the Summer 1989 issue of *Living Well with Diabetes,* the quarterly journal published by the International Diabctes Center in Minneapolis, Minnesota, Mason says that because he is black he has to recognize that he may encounter prejudices and stereotyping in his travels and be prepared for them. Once when he needed to purchase syringes he found that because of his color he was automatically suspected of being a drug user. "I could go into places, as middle-class and as old as I am," he says, "and there'd be many places that just wouldn't sell me syringes." His doctor later explained that he could always go to a hospital emergency room and get syringes. But now he also carries his doctor's phone number so he can call to request that a prescription be prepared by another doctor in the city where he's traveling. That's a good idea for anyone of any color.

Carrying a letter from your doctor explaining that you havc

diabetes and outlining your treatment needs is also a good idea. This is not just to help you get syringes or insulin or whatever else you need in an emergency, but to identify you as a diabetic in case customs inspectors notice your syringes. This is especially true for young people; we know of one young woman on a school-sponsored educational tour who was interrogated by the authorities at one border because of her syringes. They wound up believing her, but it was a very disturbing experience for her because the whole tour group was held up while she was being worked over. It was an experience that could have been avoided with a doctor's letter and plenty of diabetes identification.

In the back of our book *The Peripatetic Diabetic*, we include identification information for insulin-taking diabetics in Danish, Dutch, Finnish, French, German, Greek, Italian, Japanese, Norwegian, Portuguese, Russian, Spanish, and Swedish. Feel free to copy any of those you might need. If you can't locate the book, write to us at the SugarFree Center in Van Nuys (see Reference Section: Directory of Organizations) and tell us which ID you need; we'll be glad to run off a copy and send it to you.

Even more important than business travel, though, is the travel you do for pleasure and mind expansion. To our way of thinking, the vacation spent puttering around the house is not a vacation at all. A true vacation gets you away from home and away from the routine demands on your time and the routine worries that constantly nibble on your subconscious.

The strange thing is that if you just get away for a short time—even a weekend—you feel so restored and unstressed that it's as if you'd had a month-long holiday.

If you're nervous about handling your diabetes away from home, you might try our "expanding circle" method of travel. Make your first trip a weekend jaunt to a very nearby town or, if you live in a large city, to another part of the same city. You can pretend you're on the opposite side of the earth, but you know you can get home fast or get in touch with your doctor if there's an emergency.

When you've proved to yourself that staying in a hotel and eating all your meals out poses no problems to you or your diabetes, expand the circle farther by going someplace about five hundred miles away. Next travel all the way across the country to a place you've always wanted to visit. Then try Canada or Hawaii—both have a foreign feeling and yet pose no language or food problems.

Finally, after you've had success in these areas, go to Europe or Asia or Australia or Africa or even Antarctica, if that's your pleasure. For the truth is that a diabetic can travel anywhere that diabetics live, and, of course, that's every country on earth.

Now that you're all hyped up and ready to go, here are a few of our favorite travel tips and precautions.

- Take double quantities of all diabetes and other medical supplies that you use. It may not be easy to find them, especially overseas, and besides, who wants to spend vacation time shopping in pharmacies? If you're a belt-and-suspenders type, as June is, carry half your supplies in one place and half in another so that if you should lose a purse or piece of luggage, you'll still be covered. Then, just to be on the absolutely safe side, carry along a prescription for any medication you take. Have your doctor make this for the generic name of the drug, since the trade name may vary from country to country.

- Try to go to just one place. In the United States make it one city or national park or resort area; overseas, just one country. (A few years ago we actually went just to Rome for three weeks.) If you don't try to gulp down the whole world on a single vacation, you'll spend more time being there rather than going to a lot of different theres. You'll have more time on your feet exploring or playing than on your seat in a car or bus or train or plane. Your diabetes will show its appreciation. And if you go to only one country, you'll be able to do research ahead of time into the native cuisine to make your meals easier to figure, and more fun as well. You'll also be able to learn a few appropriate phrases in the language ("I am a diabetic." "Where is the restroom?" "Quick! Get me some sugar!").

■ Sports vacations are wonderful. Not only do you get healthful and restoring exercise while you're there, but you can also take lessons to acquire (or hone) a skill like tennis or golf or skiing that will enrich you and make your whole life healthier.

■ Two short vacations are better than one long one. You get the welcome release of a holiday at two different times of the year instead of just one. And it's true that it becomes wearisome to stay away from home for too long. June prefers vacations of one or two weeks, but if she's going overseas, she's willing to stretch it to three. Her basic rule: "I come home when all my clothes are dirty."

■ Take along two pairs of broken-in (*not* broken-down) shoes. If possible, change your shoes in the middle of the day. This helps prevent blisters. Walk and walk and walk and walk. You'll see more and get to *eat* more that way.

■ As you start your trip, make it a point to slip into what Olympic gold-medal marathon runner and attorney Frank Shorter calls his "travel mode." This means keeping relaxed and making a conscious effort not to let anything bother you. If there's a flight delay, no matter. If a crying baby is seated nearby, no matter. If someone whaps your ear with a flight bag when putting it in the overhead compartment, no matter. Remain in a semimeditative state, a king of "serene mellowness," as Shorter puts it. Getting angry and upset over the inevitable annoyances associated with travel only hurts (and raises the blood sugar of) one person: you.

■ Another Shorter travel tip is to be especially pleasant to any of the service people you deal with on a trip. He finds that courtesy is usually returned in kind and often serves to iron out potential wrinkles in your trip (and on your brow).

■ Take all the normal precautions any prudent traveler—diabetic or not—would take. For example, be sure all your basic shots are up to date. Tetanus is a particularly important one because, in case of an accident, getting a tetanus shot on top of whatever other trauma you're experiencing just exacerbates the condition. If there's a flu going around, it usually goes around everywhere, so have a shot for that unless you've had one recently. You should check with your travel agent to see what extra shots are recommended for the places you're visiting and take those as well. Any shots you take should be taken well ahead of time. If you get a reaction to any of them, you don't want it to take place on the trip. Besides, it sometimes takes a while for the immunity to set in and keep you covered. Check to find out if your health insurance covers you in foreign countries; if it doesn't, talk to your travel or insurance agent about a special short-term policy to cover you while you're traveling.

■ For foreign travel, write to the International Diabetes Federation, International Association Center, 40 Washington St., 1050 Brussels, Belgium; phone 32-2-647-44-14. They can supply you with a list of diabetes specialists in the countries you're planning to visit. Also contact Intermedic, 777 Third Ave., New York, NY 10017; phone 212-486-8974. Ask for their list of English-speaking physicians in foreign countries who are willing to treat patients for a set charge.

■ Two other handy things to take with you on a trip: a small but bright-beamed flashlight so you won't stub your toe while stumbling around strange hotel rooms in the dark looking for the bathroom or your testing materials or snacks or whatever you might need during the night for your diabetes care (this will also come in handy for reading menus in dark restaurants); and a friend or relative who understands diabetes and can help you cope with the unexpected.

■ Relax and have a good time.

Follow these rules and, indeed, the longest and most grueling of flights or bus, train, or car trips will seem shorter.

How can I get special diabetic meals on airplanes?

You can request them when you buy your tickets and the agent relays your order to the airline. If you later change your flight, you must inform the airline so that it can switch your meal order, too.

Virtually all airlines offer special diabetic trays. Once, however, when we flew United Airlines to Hawaii, the dietary-meal request slip was accidentally left on the tray. This showed that the same meal was being delivered to all those who had made these special requests for meals: diabetic, Hindu, Moslem, hypoglycemic, low calorie, low carbohydrate, low cholesterol, low fat, and low sodium. Clearly, a meal that tries to be appropriate for all of the above is not going to be totally right for any of them. And it wasn't. There was not a starch exchange to be found on the tray.

After years of trying on dozens of airlines, we've finally given up and now just take what comes. June can sort through it and pick out what she needs. After all, when immobilized on an airplane, a diabetic can eat very little anyway. It's better to concentrate not on food but rather on drinking lots of water (so you won't get dehydrated from the dry air in the cabin) and walking up and down the aisle as often as you can to keep your circulation chugging along. Drinking alcohol on a flight isn't too smart, either, since it, too, is dehydrating.

Naturally, you should bring along lots of snacks in case for some reason no food of any kind appears, or appears much later than you need it.

How can I avoid getting diarrhea when I travel in foreign countries?

Sometimes you can't. Each country has its own varieties of bacteria in the water and food. The very fact that these are different from the ones you're accustomed to causes the classic tourist problem.

As a diabetic you should, of course, do everything you possibly can to protect yourself from diarrhea. In south-of-the-border countries where *turista* is a special threat, drink only bottled water and avoid drinks containing ice. Brush your teeth using either bottled water or water you've boiled. Beware of carafes of water left on your dresser. They may well have been filled from the tap.

When all preventive measures fail, you should take some kind of antidiarrhea remedy. You'll need to consult your doctor on this, but one of our favorites is a prescription drug called Lomotil. We like it for two reasons: first, it isn't full of carbohydrates, as some of the antidiarrhea clay compounds are; and second, it's such a mite of a pill that you can swallow it with saliva if you're not near bottled water and find yourself in distress. Pepto-Bismol is also a possibility for both prevention and treatment.

Besides taking a remedy for diarrhea, try to drink a cup of broth every hour and have bananas as your fruit exchange. This restores vital salts and potassium that are lost from your system in bouts of diarrhea. An effective folk remedy is camomile tea, known in Spanish as *té de manzanilla.*

Is it all right for me to have my ears pierced? Wear acrylic nails? Have a face-lift?

It seemed to be a good idea to group all these appearance-enhancing questions together since they have basically the same answer.

We first became aware of the ear-piercing problem when Barbara had hers pierced. She was made to sign a consent slip stating that she didn't have diabetes. Since she isn't diabetic, signing it posed no problem, but it did set her to thinking that it didn't seem fair to keep diabetics from getting their ears pierced if they wanted to. We checked with some of our experts.

Richard K. Bernstein, diabetic diabetologist of Mamaroneck, New York, was of the opinion that the restriction made sense because the vast majority of diabetics are in such poor control that it would be an infection risk for them.

Diana Guthrie, a diabetes nurse specialist, had a more positive approach: "So long as your blood sugars are normalized or near normalized, there should be no hesitation whatsoever in getting your ears pierced if the proper precautions that are taken for everybody else are taken for you."

Assuming you take care of this risk factor, you're left with only the dilemma of whether to sign the paper saying that you're *not* diabetic. Since the ear-piercing brigade is probably having you sign only to protect itself in the event of an infection, it would seem that all you're doing is denying yourself legal recourse if something should go wrong. But whether to sign is a moral question rather than a diabetic one, and we aren't the best source of the answer.

The reason we brought up the question of acrylic nails is that we know diabetics are more susceptible to nail fungus than others. Attaching these nails might therefore cause fungus to develop or spread. Diana Guthrie again set our minds at ease. She explains: "Glued-on nails do not enhance the development of fungal infections so long as careful hand-washing techniques are routinely instituted and the fungal organism is not overwhelmingly present." One of our SugarFree employees, Melanie Epperson, who also has her own nail business, echoes this sentiment. She has several diabetic clients who have acrylic nails, and not one has ever had a problem with them.

And now we get to the biggie—a face-lift. We won't debate

here the advisability of cosmetic surgery (which is questionable unless the surgery is done to correct something like a cleft palate or to repair the ravages of an accident). If you do decide, for whatever personal reasons, that you would like to have a face-lift, the question is, Should your diabetes stand in your way? Again we hear good news from Diana Guthrie: "The advisability of anyone getting a face-lift or other cosmetic surgery is the same as for any surgical procedure. If someone has diabetes and it is *under control,* they probably will heal faster and better than even the nondiabetic. There should be no hesitation to do surgical procedures, so long as the service of a knowledgeable physician is available to manage the diabetes before, during, and after the procedure." Lois Jovanovic-Peterson agrees. This goes along with her philosophy that diabetics who are in control can do virtually anything they'd do if they weren't diabetic.

So the answer to all of the above (and all of life) is yes, if your diabetes is *under control.*

Is it all right for me to use generic drugs?

Before we answer that, we'd like you to have an understanding of what generic drugs are. We'd long been confused about them ourselves, so we asked Mike Voelker, Pharm. D., our SugarFree Centers Director of Pharmacy Services, to explain them. The first thing we found out surprised us: pharmacies actually make a greater percentage of profit on generics than on brand names, so if your pharmacist discourages you from purchasing a certain generic, he's doing it for professional reasons and not out of some sordid profit motive.

Mike further explains that generic drugs (drugs not protected by trademark) are in demand today for many valid reasons. First, insurance companies and other health-cost payment systems are encouraging their members to use generic drugs by offering people a lower copayment if they do. Second, the FDA is shortening the time period for trade-name drugs to become ge-

neric. And third, over the next three to four years, as the federal
government (Medicare) phases in payments for prescription
drugs (just as the state of California now does with its Medi-Cal
drug program), it will probably demand that generic medications
be provided whenever possible.

For the above reasons, it's safe to say that generics are here
to stay. But . . . buyer, beware! Some warnings are in order.
Brand-name drugs and their generic forms are not necessarily
identical. Switching to a generic without proper precautions may
cause serious problems. To understand the possible difficulties,
you have to understand what generic drugs are and how they're
made.

A generic drug has exactly the same amount of the active
ingredient as the trade-name product. The active ingredient by
weight, however, makes up only a fraction of the total weight of
the tablet or capsule. For example, a Lanoxin 0.25 mg tablet
weighs about 1.5 mg, but the active ingredient (Digoxin) makes
up only about 10 percent of the total weight of the tablet. The
other 90 percent comprises what pharmacists call excipients—
fillers, binding agents, coloring, etc. It is these extra ingredients
that very often determine how much of the active drug is absorbed into the bloodstream and how quickly. In some cases
more drug is absorbed and in other cases less. This difference
can be critical, depending on the type of drug you're using.

With the following classes of drugs, you and your doctor
and pharmacist must be extremely careful when changing to the
generic form:

- cardiovascular drugs (Digoxin, Inderal, etc.)
- hormone and related drugs (Premarin)
- psychotherapeutic drugs (Thorazine, Elavil, etc.)
- anticonvulsants (Dilantin)
- oral hypoglycemics (Orinase, Diabenese, etc.)

A diabetic, for example, can switch from the trade-name Orinase to the generic tolbutamide, but you should always ask your physician first. When the switch is made, you must be very diligent about testing for hyper- or hypoglycemia so you can determine whether the generic is being absorbed in the same way as the trade-name pill. Then, once you have successfully switched, you have to make sure you are always provided with that particular brand of generic, because *generics also differ from brand to brand.* This is another complication, which means that only those in the know can protect themselves from drug overdose or underdose.

With classes of drugs not on the above list, such as antibiotics and analgesics, it is perfectly okay to switch to a generic brand without any special monitoring.

The final word on generics, then, is to go ahead and enjoy the savings they offer, but make sure that you, your physician, and your pharmacist work as a team to ensure their safe and efficacious use.

For
Insulin-Dependent
Diabetics (Type I)

. . . .

June has always felt that diabetics who take insulin are the real thing. In fact, in some of her more resentful moments, she sometimes refers to those who can make it on diet and exercise alone or on diet, exercise, and pills as "those fake diabetics." Of course, she knows in her heart that it's not true. All diabetics are the real thing and have real problems.

And yet even the non-insulin-takers themselves realize they have it a lot easier. To their minds the ultimate horror is often the idea of having to go onto the needle—a "horror" that insulin-dependents already live with.

As June says of herself and her fellow needle jockeys, "You've got to admit that we're the ones who are most involved with diabetes. In fact, it's never out of our minds (and it had better not be!).We have the needle and the daily injections; the constant lookout for insulin shock; the need to have something sugary available at all times; the problem of keeping medical supplies in stock; the expense of needles, insulin, and syringes; the precise food requirements, with eating too little as big a mistake as eating too much; the necessity of stuffing some therapeutic food down for insulin's sake when you're not even hungry; the inevitable snacks between meals and at bedtime; the incomprehensions of family, coworkers, and acquaintances; the isolation and apartness caused by being different."

Because of all this, insulin takers develop a special kinship with one another. All barriers are broken down. Seventy-year-olds communicate easily with eighteen-year-olds, sharing their problems and their solutions, trading information, and gaining understanding of one another and themselves in the process. It's a close-knit subculture in which every member will leap forward to help the other in time of trouble. It's almost like a secret society—"the Diabetic Mafia," as Barbara calls it.

In this section we'll share the experiences and discoveries of the members of our Diabetic Mafia family in hopes that we can put a contract on your problems and send them to the bottom of the East River.

What is insulin?

Insulin, as we mentioned earlier, is the hormone that helps the body cells take up sugar from the blood. As a Type I diabetic, you must inject insulin to replace your body's lack of the hormone. The amount to be injected every day depends on whether your body is producing none or only a small amount. If it is producing none, your injections are a substitute for your own insulin; if it is producing some, you have to augment your own insulin with injections. Your physician will determine how much insulin you need and which kinds.

There are two kinds of insulin: fast-acting and slow-acting. Fast-acting insulin is called Regular insulin or Semi-lente. It begins acting in about half an hour and lasts approximately one to five hours. The slow-acting insulins are divided into two types: intermediate-acting and long-acting. Intermediate-acting insulins are called NPH and Lente. These begin acting in about an hour and a half and last approximately twelve to twenty-four hours.

Long-acting insulins are called Ultralente and PZI. These begin to take effect in four to six hours and can last up to thirty-six hours. Most diabetics take a combination of fast-acting and inter- mediate- or long-acting insulins.

Injectable insulins come in bottles of ten cubic centimeters each. Fast-acting insulin is clear, and slow-acting is cloudy. In- sulin is measured in units. All insulin sold in the United States is of the same concentration: U100, which means that there are one hundred units of insulin in each cubic centimeter. So a ten-cubic centimeter bottle would contain one thousand units of insulin. If your dosage of insulin is ten units a day, then a bottle of insulin will last you about one hundred days. We say *about*, because you can't get the last couple of drops out of the bottle.

The insulins sold in the United States are manufactured by three major companies: Lilly, Squibb-Novo, and Nordisk. All insulin used to be made from the pancreas of pigs and steers. Though many people still use animal insulin, the new insulins made in laboratories by changing pork insulin to human insulin (Squibb-Novo, Nordisk) or by DNA technology (Lilly) are pre- ferred. Since these semisynthetic and synthetic human insulins are identical to the body's own, they do not cause antibodies or allergic reactions, and they are absorbed more quickly. Human insulins are extremely pure (99.999 percent) compared with the animal insulins of the past. And even the newer animal insulins called "purified" are 99.99 percent pure. So if you must take insulin, at least you know that it can be of unimpeachable quality.

Most physicians think everyone should now use human in- sulin. Oddly enough, though, not all old-time diabetics can suc- cessfully switch to human insulin and maintain the same control they had with animal insulin. There are also diabetics who can- not afford to change from the old beef-pork combination because it is much less expensive than human or purified pork. (We hope that's not you.)

Insulins now have such great variety—there are even some that are premixed as 70 percent intermediate-acting and 30 percent fast-acting—that you must make absolutely certain when you go shopping that you're getting exactly what your doctor prescribed and even the same brand he prescribed. Take the empty bottle with you. Another tip: keep a backup supply of at least one bottle, as not all pharmacies stock all varieties of insulin, and you may dash out to replace your vial only to find that your pharmacy has none.

Why can't I just take my insulin in a pill?

Insulin is a protein, and if it were delivered in pill form, the stomach would digest it the way it would a hamburger; you'd get no benefit from it. Researchers are now working on encapsulating insulin in a substance that would allow it to pass through the stomach without being digested and then be released in the intestine.

Since people don't like to have to inject insulin, many other possibilities have been and are being worked on. These include insulin suppositories and nasal spray. Insulin suppositories were developed in Israel but were never distributed widely, probably because they would not be likely to gain any more popular acceptance than injections. Nasal spray has so far not been shown to absorb evenly. Colds could also pose a problem. Actually, nasal insulin was never intended to totally replace injected insulin but only to reduce the number of injections required and to improve control. There is another method called the insulin patch, but insulin molecules proved to be too large to pass through the skin.

Once you start taking insulin, do you have to take it for the rest of you life?

If you're a Type I diabetic, yes, you're probably stuck (!) with it. Occasionally after children or young people are first diagnosed and start using insulin, there comes a honeymoon period. The disease seems to fade away, they can stop taking insulin, and their family believes a miracle has occurred and they are cured. Not so. Like all honeymoons, the diabetes honeymoon eventually comes to an end, and insulin injections must begin again. (But enjoy it while it lasts.)

Sometimes if you're a Type II diabetic you may be on insulin only until you get your weight down.

Also, diabetics who aren't normally on insulin may have to take it when they're sick or have an infection or are pregnant. When they're well again, or the baby is delivered, they can stop.

Where and how do I inject insulin?

Insulin can be injected into the arm, abdomen, buttocks, or thigh. To make sure you stay within the proper area of each of these sites, you can order the pamphlet *Site Selection and Rotation* from Becton Dickinson Consumer Products, Franklin Lakes, NJ 07417-1883.

It's very important to rotate your injections within each area, because there are differences in the speed with which insulin is absorbed, depending on where it is injected. Injection in the abdomen is fastest—30 to 50 percent faster than in other areas; next fastest are arms and legs. The usual lag time for the abdomen is 30 to 40 minutes, while in the arm or leg the time lag is usually around 40 to 50 minutes. Insulin also acts faster in places that are lean rather than fat. According to Dr. Jay S. Skyler, professor of medicine, pediatrics, and psychology at the University of Miami School of Medicine, it is preferable to inject all before-meal shots of regular insulin into the abdomen for faster action. This will help prevent post-meal blood sugar from being too high.

A few more tricks to speed up the action of regular insulin include taking a warm shower or placing a hot washcloth over the injection site. The warmer the skin temperature is, the faster the insulin is absorbed. Exercising an area into which insulin has been injected also speeds up the action. For example, it is recommended that you avoid injecting it into your legs and arms before playing tennis, and avoid injecting it into your thighs if you are going to run or jog.

Dr. Skyler, in a speech at the 1989 Annual Meeting of the American Association of Diabetes Educators, also pointed out that you cannot count on insulin absorbing at the same rate after each injection. In fact, within the same individual, absorption time has an average difference of 25 percent. But the smaller the dose, the better the action. That's one more advantage to multiple injections.

Your doctor or the nurse who teaches you the injection technique will give you complete instructions about when to take your doses of insulin. Since fast-acting insulins begin to work in about a half hour, you are usually instructed to take the shot a half hour before eating.

Many people, like June, judge by their blood sugar. If it is too much above normal before a meal (she takes regular insulin before each meal), she will postpone her meal by as much as an hour so that the insulin will have started to bring her blood sugar down before she eats food. If her blood sugar is on the low side before a meal, she will eat without waiting even the half hour.

In many instances, of course, you cannot follow an ideal timing schedule because of the unpredictable nature of life. One morning you may oversleep, be in a hurry to get to work, and take your shot five minutes before breakfast. Another morning you may get an unexpected telephone call after the injection and delay breakfast for three-quarters of an hour. We've heard of even stranger variations from diabetics, like the man who told us, "Lots of times I eat breakfast and take my injection after I'm finished."

In the final analysis you have to work out your own best timing with your doctor so that you can keep your blood sugar and your lifestyle as close to normal as humanly possible.

How can I get over my fear of the needle?

First of all, don't feel you're more cowardly than anyone else. We've never met any people who enjoyed sticking themselves with a needle. (And in fact, we'd rather not meet any.) We have met several, though, who swore they'd never be able to do it, but when the golden moment arrived they found they could, as Lady Macbeth put it, screw their courage to the sticking place.

Most insulin-dependent diabetics who inject themselves—and many do it two or three times a day for better management—get so used to it that it's fairly routine. (We won't give you the nonsense that "it becomes like brushing your teeth.")

Sometimes people can inject themselves for years without being bothered by it. Then suddenly they begin building up dread again. If you haven't yet conquered your fear or if you find it suddenly reappearing, here's what you can do about it.

- If you have the habit of worrying about the injection and how much it's going to hurt, instead picture yourself doing it easily and without pain. Positive thinking brings about positive results.

- If you've been having someone else give you shots, start giving them yourself. Not only is this necessary in case of emergencies, but you'll reinforce your feelings of competence. You may even discover that it hurts less when you do it yourself. We tend to tense our muscles when someone else is taking a poke at us.

- Relax. Those tense muscles we just mentioned not only make the shot hurt more but can also cause bruising. (And getting bruises is not a way to make yourself fear the needle less.)

- June found that when she switched from one to three shots a day, and then later on to five, an amazing change took place: she lost all dread of the needle. This may sound ridiculous, but it's true. Our explanation is that the more often you do it, the less time you'll have to build up a wall of worry. You inject your insulin as calmly as you'd do any other daily task.

A dividend you get from mastering your insulin injections is a feeling of power, an "If I can do this, I can do anything" feeling. You'll find you become a stronger person in every way.

Now, having given you this pep talk to make you positively panting with eagerness to stick yourself with a needle, we'll deliver the news that you don't have to if you don't want to. Modern technology strikes again to make diabetes self-care easier and less traumatic.

The Insuflon. A partial solution to the constant jabbing yourself with needles is a recent innovation from Sweden called the Insuflon. It has been tested there for four years and is used by 12 percent of the Type I diabetics in Scandinavia. The Insuflon is a short, soft, paper-thin tube that is inserted in the abdomen with a needle, which is removed immediately after insertion. The tube remains in place for a recommended three to five days and all shots are given through its resealable opening. This allows you to have one skin puncture for that entire period of time instead of the usual two or three a day.

Pat Ockel, the manager of our Del Mar SugarFree Center, wore an Insuflon for a few days and recommended it to June, who bruises and bleeds easily when taking her three or four shots of regular insulin each day—all in the abdomen for fast absorption. The insertion needle, which is one-quarter of an inch longer than the usual needle, is admittedly a bit intimidating. But with Pat's guidance, June wore it for a whole week—two days longer than the recommended time. It worked beautifully for her. She considered it one of the least painful and easiest methods she's tried: "While I was wearing it, I was amazed to find I couldn't feel it at all."

When June removed the Insuflon, there was only a tiny red dot at the injection site, which quickly disappeared. She suggests that anyone starting on the Insuflon might need a brief lesson from a trained health professional. It's such a new concept that even experienced needle users need some guidance the first time around. Insuflons come in boxes of four and ten (SugarFree Centers also sell them individually for those wanting to try them out.) They cost approximately $11 each, $39.95 for a box of four, or $85 for a box of ten. For further information call Diabetes Centers, Inc., 800-848-0614 (address: 13911 Ridgedale Dr., Ste. 250, Minneapolis, Minnesota 55343).

What is an automatic injector?

An automatic injector takes a loaded syringe and shoots it into you so quickly that you hardly know it happened. It gives you perfect injection technique, and since you don't even see the needle in the device, it does a lot toward keeping you relaxed. Not only do these devices eliminate the fear and pain, but you can reach a lot of new injection territory and reach it with one hand—especially important for parents of small children, for whom the statement "This hurts me more than it does you" is often true. When a parent uses one of these devices, everybody is happier. People with arthritis or other dexterity problems also find these a boon. But the greatest advantage of automatic injectors is that they facilitate the multiple injections many people need to keep their diabetes under control and help them avoid complications.

The currently available injectors include the Injectomatic (Sherwood Medical), the Autojector and the Diamatic (Ulster Scientific), the Inject-Ease (Palco), and the Instaject II (Jordan Enterprises). Some are pictured on page 142. The prices range from around $20 up to $140, with most falling between $30 and $50. Most injectors can accommodate all sizes and brands of syringes. (Note: The Injectomatic is usable only with Monoject syringes, which isn't too surprising since Sherwood makes both.)

After the injector zaps in the needle, you press the syringe plunger to release the insulin. (With the Autojector and its luxurious variation, the Diamatic, the insulin is released automatically.)

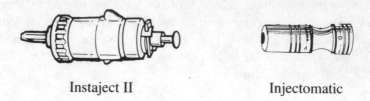

Instaject II   Injectomatic

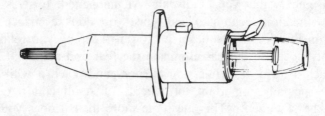

Inject-Ease

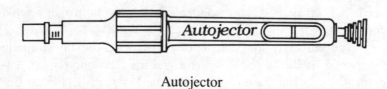

Autojector

Automatic injectors.

Even with an automatic injector, though, it's true you're still using a needle, and if needles are intrinsically horrifying to you, there is yet another alternative.

What is a jet injector?

With a jet injector you can totally rid yourself of needles. The insulin itself is shot in with jetlike speed so that all you feel is something like snapping your finger against your skin. You can mix insulins in the jets just as you can with needles. June is such a fanatic for control, though, that she takes her regular and her long-acting insulins in two different jets and at two different sites (abdomen for regular; elsewhere for long-acting).

But the greatest advantage of jet injectors is not the fact that you're freed from needles. It's the improved control with less insulin that many people achieve. With needles, sometimes the insulin pools at the injection site after you inject it. (This is called "depoting" in the trade.) When this happens with a mixed dose of insulin, it can slow down the action of the regular so you don't get its effect when you need it. It can also happen that the insulin sitting in its pool isn't absorbed as quickly as it should be to keep you in control, and then, *whammo*, it's released later on when you don't need it, and your blood sugar plummets.

Some complain that jet injectors sometimes make bruises, but then so do needles. Everyone complains about the price. They're now close to eight hundred dollars, but that's not too surprising when you realize how complex they are. Over the years you gradually make up the price in not having to buy syringes, but it is a big initial hit.

Fortunately, more and more insurance companies are covering jet injectors when prescribed by a physician. You often can submit a prior-approval form to your insurance company so you'll know in advance if they'll pay, and thus avoid playing financial roulette. Insurance companies are probably beginning to cover jet injectors because they realize that anything that will encourage people to take more injections and stay in better control (and out of hospitals) is a good investment.

Now, having sung the praises of automatic injectors and jets loud and long, we must quickly add that before you get either, you must tough it out and learn how to inject with a syringe—

and always keep them handy—because you never know when you may accidentally drop your injector off the back of your yacht. This actually happened to one man we know. He would have been high and dry on his yacht without his backup syringes.

Incidentally, because jet-injector manufacturers want to show that their instruments are easy enough for a child to use, their ads usually show children injecting. One time a grown-up man came into the SugarFree Center and wistfully inquired, "Are those jet injectors just for kids? I sure would love to have one."

While they're not *just* for kids, a bright independent kid can quickly master one. A prime example is one eleven-year-old we know, George Anderson III, who became so adept that he could load his Medi-Jector in the two minutes it took to complete his blood-sugar test. George's mother, who wisely lets George take charge of his own therapy, didn't really concentrate on the training in the jet lessons because George proved so adept. Then George got quite ill with a virus. He couldn't use the jet, and his mother had to resort to using the needle on him. Needless (needleless!) to say, having to get stuck was a great incentive for George to get well fast. And his first job upon recovery was to teach his mother the art and science of jet injection.

Is the insulin-infusion pump I've heard about another way of getting off needles?

You could say that, but really the most important advantage of a pump is that it's possible to achieve better control with it. Even people who've had trouble keeping their blood sugar normal for years find that a pump can bring it under control—and keep it there!

The insulin-infusion pump is another of the exciting advances in the wonderful world of modern diabetes therapies. In just the last few years pumps have gone from primitive, awkward, and semiunpredictable instruments to small, efficient, reliable, and highly sophisticated marvels of technology. They now are compact and sturdy, weigh only around three ounces, and are battery operated, splashproof, and programmable.

You wear the pump on a belt or strapped to your leg or actually anywhere it's convenient. The pump then delivers regular insulin at specific intervals to take care of your metabolic needs. The insulin travels through a slender, flexible tube and enters your body via a needle or, better still, a cannula (a tiny plastic tube) that is inserted under your skin at any normal injection site, usually the abdominal area. The needle or cannula stays in place for one to three days and then is rotated to a different spot, just as you change injection sites when using syringes and needles.

When it's time for a meal, you press a button to release the appropriate amount of regular insulin to cover the meal. Most pump wearers figure their mealtime insulin needs by counting carbohydrates.

Their programmability is one of the most valuable features of modern pumps. For example, people who inject long-acting insulin often get low blood sugar in the middle of the night and then their blood sugar goes up in the very early morning (a condition known as the dawn phenomenon). The pump wearer can program the pump to deliver less insulin during the period when blood sugar is likely to be down and more insulin for the dawn blood-sugar rise.

You have to work very closely with your diabetes health-care team during the period when you're finding out what your body's metabolic requirements are for insulin, the daily fluctuations of your blood sugar, and how insulin sensitive or insulin resistant you are in order to discover how much insulin will cover how many grams of carbohydrate for you. But after all that's worked out, you can have amazing control and amazing flexibility in your lifestyle and mealtimes.

The best way for you to understand what pump wearing is like is to hear it from a pump wearer. Pat Ockel really never had any desire to go onto a pump. She went onto one initially to participate in a pump study for which volunteers were needed but then . . . well, let's let Pat tell her own tale.

I've been on an insulin-infusion pump for two and a half years, the last two on a MiniMed. I got my MiniMed just before I went on an African safari in June 1987. It was one of the smallest pumps available; at that time it was the only one that was splash-proof and could get wet without being harmed; it had the largest reservoir [it carries three hundred units of insulin]; and it worked off of three small batteries that could be found at most drugstores, even in Africa.

It took me about a year and a half to decide if I really wanted to be on a pump. After all, I had normal A_1C's on four shots a day with syringes. The idea of having a needle in me twenty-four hours a day and having to carry a little box around wasn't a big thrill, though the idea of flexible mealtimes really appealed to me, especially because at the SugarFree Center it wasn't always convenient to eat right at noon when everybody seems to rush in, and I was always having to down Dextrosol glucose tablets to keep going.

When MiniMed introduced the Sof-set, that made me decide I'd like to try a pump, since if you didn't need a needle inserted in you all the time, the pump wouldn't be much of a problem. A Sof-set has the needle enclosed in a soft plastic tube, and after you insert it, you pull out the needle and only the soft tube remains. This makes Sof-sets much more comfortable, because you can use them in the legs or your hip and you don't have to worry about having the needle hurt when you do heavy exercise or hit it with your purse or bump somebody.

After I got my MiniMed pump, my husband said that my moods really smoothed out compared to when I was on shots. (I wasn't aware that I had these mood swings when I used syringes, but apparently they were quite noticeable to him.) Also, I haven't had any bad reactions the way I used to with syringes. A misconception I had about pumps was that once you put it on you couldn't take it off. That's not true! If you want to go to the beach for the day, you can easily take it off and use syringes that day. In fact, it's not a bad idea to take it off occasionally, because some people actually forget how to take shots with a syringe and would be in trouble if something went wrong with their pump. The strange thing is that once you start wearing a pump with a Sof-set you actually aren't aware that it's there. And it certainly makes it convenient for eating at restaurants when you just pull the pump out and take your dose right at the table.

Of course, having a pump doesn't make you any less responsible for your diabetes. You still have to do as many blood-sugar tests—if not more—so you can tell the pump what to do according to your blood-sugar level. And it does take more learning to enjoy the freedom the pump gives you with your eating. For example, you have to learn the specific carbohydrate value of foods.

Since I used to scorn the pump, everybody at the SugarFree Center was amazed when I went onto one—and I've been amazed at how happy I've been on it.

For further information on pumps, write or call:

MiniMed Technologies (MiniMed pump, Sof-set), 12744 San Fernando Rd., Sylmar, CA 91342, 800-843-6687 (nationwide, except California), 800-826-2099 (California).

CPI/Lilly (Betatron), 4100 N. Hamline Ave., St. Paul, MN 55112, 800-328-9588.

Medical Electronics USA (Medix), 1010 Park St., Peekskill, NY 10566, 914-737-1646.

What if I forget to take my insulin injection?

At least you'll know you're not obsessed with your disease. But if this happens more than once in a great while, you'll need to devise some kind of reminder system, like a nagging husband, wife, or parent. If you have small children, you can give them a penny each time you take the shot. (They'll never forget, but don't let them con you into taking your shot twice.) When it does dawn on you that you forgot your shot, take your blood sugar and see what's happening. Call your doctor, who can probably help you decide how much insulin to take, if any. Much depends on what kind of insulin you take and how many shots a day you take, so general advice is of no help.

Sometimes the problem is even worse. It's remembering whether or not you took the insulin. Then you have to worry about getting a double dose or no dose at all. If you use diposable needles (doesn't everyone?), you can look into the wastebasket and find out. If you're at a total loss and can't figure out whether you did or didn't, the safer course is not to take a shot. Think how tough it would be and how much time it would take to eat all the extra food the double injection would require, not to mention the weight it would put on. There's no doubt that a good memory is a help to a diabetic.

When I'm sick and can't eat, do I stop taking insulin?

That's a good question, as politicians being interviewed by reporters like to say. The answer is no, no, a thousand times no. If you have severe nausea and vomiting and can't keep anything down, you can sometimes reduce your normal daily insulin dose by one-half or two-thirds (if your blood sugars are normal). But more often when you're sick, your blood sugar goes up and you need more insulin, not less. (Illness makes insulin less effective.) Sometimes your doctor (keep in touch when you're sick) will prescribe additional shots of regular (fast-acting) insulin before each meal.

For sick days when you can't eat solid food, the usual recommendation is to sip ginger ale (to control nausea and to satisfy your insulin) and to drink clear broth or fruit juices every hour.

Whenever you're sick, especially with the flu, a cold, an injury, or an infection, you have to watch your diabetes more closely. Take your blood sugar every few hours. If it's over 240, check your urine for ketones. If ketones appear, call your doctor immediately. Blood-sugar levels can go very high during illness, and your doctor can help you bring them down safely. But don't just sit there—or lie there—and do nothing. This is not a situation you can safely ignore.

Do insulin syringes and needles require a prescription?

This one's a real puzzler. The answer is that they do and they don't. In California, for example, most pharmacists require only the diabetic's signature, not the doctor's. Some, however, insist on a doctor's prescription. The laws vary from state to state, and the interpretation of the laws varies from pharmacy to pharmacy.

We've never tried purchasing this equipment out of state or overseas, but June always carries a doctor's prescription in case the occasion should ever arise.

Do I need to clean the skin with alcohol before I inject?

We hate to advocate unhygienic practices, but we also hate for you to get all agitated and upset if you don't have any alcohol or an alcohol swab along when you need to take a shot.

For what it's worth, June never cleans the injection site with alcohol—unless, of course, she hasn't been able to bathe on a daily basis. One doctor told us there was a British study in which they gave five thousand injections using alcohol and five thousand without. There were only five infections in the whole lot, and all those were in cases where alcohol had been used! (The doctor laughed and said maybe the alcohol irritated the bacteria and stirred them into action.)

How do I take care of my bottles of insulin?

Bottles is the correct word, because you should have more than one on hand. The backup supply should be kept in the refrigerator (not in the coldest part, where it might freeze, and certainly not in the freezer compartment). The bottle you're using (or bottles, if you use more than one kind) should stay at room temperature and be conveniently placed in whatever room you use to take your shots. Don't keep your opened bottles refrigerated. Not only is this unnecessary, but cold insulin causes more pain when injected and does not absorb as well. Insulin remains stable up to three months without refrigeration. Always write the date you opened it on the side of the bottle.

You should, by the way, always watch the expiration date on your insulin. If you use it after that date it may not be as effective. For that reason, you can't stock up on huge quantities of insulin when you find it on sale. That's not a good idea anyway, as you might change insulins.

When June finds herself out of control, the first thing she checks is the date on the insulin she's using. If the insulin is slightly out of date, she throws it away hastily. (Although she admits it usually turns out that the insulin was not at fault.)

It's perfectly okay to carry your insulin in your purse or pocket (in a protective case of some kind) when you're not going to be taking your injection at home. Insulin is pretty hardy stuff. You just have to be careful not to freeze it or expose it to high temperatures (above one hundred degrees Fahrenheit).

When traveling you don't have to worry about keeping your insulin refrigerated, but you do have to worry about where to keep it. In airplanes, don't put your insulin in the luggage you check. Keep it in your pocket, purse, or hand luggage, both because the cargo hold may be too cold and because your luggage may get lost along the way. If you're traveling by automobile, don't leave your insulin in a closed car in the hot sun because the temperature can rise to damaging heights.

Many people like to buy an insulated carrying case for insulin, especially if they're planning a trip to an extremely hot or cold climate. The safest container, which works both ways, is also unfortunately the largest. It's the Medicool, which has a prerefrigeratable section that will keep insulin cool even in a hundred-degree oven. Unrefrigerated, the same section keeps insulin from freezing. The Dia-Pod also does double duty. It is an ultralight holder made of the tiniest of foam beads for maximum insulation. And the Insul-Tote is a foam-insulated bag that includes a refreezable refrigerant. New kinds of cases are constantly appearing, so watch for the one that suits you. These sorts of products can be purchased at most diabetes supply centers.

What causes those lumps that I sometimes get after a shot?

It could be that you've injected too frequently in the same place or that you're allergic to the kind of insulin you're using—or both. Try to be more conscientious about rotating the injection site. If the lumps continue to appear, tell your doctor, who may change the type of insulin you're using.

Some people get skin indentations or depressions instead of lumps. These are caused by losing fat wherever you inject insulin (fat atrophy). The correction for both problems, if you aren't on human insulin now, is often to change to human.

Can I get along on one shot of intermediate-acting insulin a day?

Almost definitely not. The therapeutic life of human NPH (the length of time it controls blood sugar) is only twelve to fourteen hours. The other intermediate-acting insulin, Lente, controls for only fourteen to sixteen hours. You can see that using only one shot of either of these insulins would leave you uncovered for a lot of time during a twenty-four-hour period. Not only that, but taking it in one shot would mean that the insulin would peak once, possibly at a time when you very likely wouldn't have planned to have your main meal. You'd have to feed your insulin when it demanded it and then not be able to eat when you (and everyone else) wanted to. So not only is one shot bad therapy, it makes for a rigid and unpleasant life.

Dr. Lois Jovanovic-Peterson does admit that people who still have some pancreatic function can get along on only one shot of NPH. If you always have normal fasting blood sugars on the one-shot-a-day plan, you are among the few lucky ones who can do it. Dr. Jovanovic-Peterson emphasizes, though, that the vast majority of Type I diabetics who have no pancreatic function can't possibly have good control with one shot of NPH a day—no matter how much they'd love to do it. `

You keep talking about taking all those injections to keep blood sugar normal. How do I handle it when I'm out at restaurants?

It's not all that difficult, thanks to the many helpful devices the diabeticization of America has produced.

You can load your syringe at home and carry it in a PDI (predrawn insulin) case, which was invented by a diabetic who needed it himself. (This is how practical diabetes products are often created.) The case is slim and unobtrusive, yet it's large enough to hold two predrawn syringes. Your syringe sits cozily in foam so the insulin can't be released accidentally. In the restaurant restroom or even in the car prior to entering the restaurant, it's quick and easy to take your shot even if the lighting isn't bright enough for measuring your insulin.

Another new development that's particularly handy for injecting away from home is the NovolinPen. As you might surmise from the name, it looks like a pen. You load it with a cartridge of Novolin regular, NPH, or 70/30 (70 percent NPH, 30 percent regular). Each cartridge contains 150 units of insulin. You can dial in the number of units you want to take (from 2 to 36 in 2-unit increments) and shoot it in. You change the disposable needle at the end of the pen as needed.

We've heard that other pen injectors are in the works from Ulster Scientific (Accupen) and Nordisk. By the time you read this they may be on the market.

How do I adjust my insulin when I fly and change time zones?

That depends strictly on your insulin schedule, what kind of insulin you take, and how many shots a day you require. And there's more than one method for calculating the adjustments.

To give you a basic understanding of the problem, remember that time change occurs only when you fly east or west, not north or south. Flying from west to east, your day is shortened. Flying from east to west, it is lengthened. So when flying east, you lower your dosage; when flying west, you increase it. *But* if the change is not more than four hours, you don't need to take any special action. Likewise, if your total insulin dose is small—only ten or fifteen units—you can probably get by without any change.

If you monitor your blood sugar frequently, you can stay out of trouble and in control, no matter what. Knowing how to adjust insulin according to blood sugar and giving yourself supplements of regular insulin makes the whole thing easy. Otherwise, discuss your insulin program with your physician or nurse educator. First prepare yourself if you can by reading about the different ways to handle the situation. Read *The Joslin Diabetes Manual* or *Controlling Diabetes the Easy Way* by Stanley Mirsky (see Recommended Reading) or any other basic diabetes-education book that covers the subject.

Airborne-injection tip: When you take an insulin injection in a plane, do not inject air into the bottle. If you do, because of the difference in air pressure the plunger will fight you and make it difficult to measure accurately.

Is it all right to have low blood sugar?

No. Low blood sugar—or insulin reaction, as low blood sugar is often called—can be very hazardous for a diabetic, because you become irritable, befuddled, uncoordinated, and, in extreme cases, unconscious. Automobile accidents are not the only possible danger. One of our friends fell in his swimming pool when he blacked out during an insulin reaction and was lucky enough to be awakened by the water and make it to the side and climb out. Maybe you read the story of Candy Sangster, who became unconscious during a weekend at home alone. She was saved by her dog, Jet, who went outside and barked until the neighbors decided to dial 911. Jet, a six-year-old Doberman, was named the Ken-L-Ration Dog Hero of the Year in 1986 for his dramatic life-saving exploit. So if you don't own a dog, don't be lax about hypoglycemia.

The most logical way to check to see if you're having an insulin reaction is to take your blood sugar. You should also learn to recognize the characteristic physical and/or mental changes that take place.

If your blood sugar is dropping fast: shakiness, sweating, dizziness, poor coordination, palpitations, hunger, irritability, and nausea.

If your blood sugar is dropping slowly: slurred speech, blurred vision, confusion. You may be so confused, in fact, that you don't realize you're having a reaction.

If you should find yourself without your blood-testing supplies (tsk!), you can also check your pulse. During a reaction, your pulse will ordinarily be one-third higher than your resting pulse. (To be able to do this you have to learn what your resting pulse is. To do this, take it several times when you're sitting around relaxed and doing nothing.)

As people get older, especially if they haven't had good control of their diabetes over the years, their signals of low blood sugar sometimes diminish as a result of autonomic neuropathy. Strangely enough, your signals can also diminish because of good control. When people in good control get low blood sugar, they may be going from only around 100 to the 30s and 40s, so they don't get the dramatic signals that people plunging there from the 200s do. (Note: This is *not* a recommendation that you keep your blood sugar high so you'll get better signals of low blood sugar.)

Why do I sometimes feel as if I'm having an insulin reaction when my blood sugar is normal?

It could be that physical or psychological factors unrelated to your diabetes are making you feel strange. But we have talked to several diabetics who maintain that they feel better with high blood sugar and that when it's normal they feel as if they're hypoglycemic.

Most of those who experience this phenomenon have been running around for quite a while with high blood sugar, either because they weren't testing their blood sugar and didn't realize how high it was or because they'd just been sloppy in their diabetes care. You know the song "I've Been Down So Long It Feels Like Up to Me"? Well, these diabetics have been up so long it feels like normal to them. Consequently, when they start bringing their blood sugar down to where it should be, they feel unnatural. It's almost like coming off a drug.

But if you stick to it and keep your blood sugar in the normal range, before long you'll feel right only when your blood sugar's right.

What do I do for an insulin reaction?

You eat or drink something sweet that will bring your blood sugar up fast. (This always confuses nondiabetics, who are convinced that diabetics can *never* have anything sugary and resist giving them what they need.) Most lists of what to eat for insulin reactions have been the same for years—and still are. They include a half glass of orange juice, sugar cubes, three or four Lifesavers, a half cup of Coke or Pepsi, two tablespoons of raisins, etc. We've never understood how anyone could conceive of some of these items as handy to carry in your purse or pocket at all times. And we particularly don't fathom the magic of orange juice. It's actually low on the Carbohydrate Glycemic Index (46).

What you need in a low-blood-sugar emergency—and it

should be treated as an emergency—is something quick and easy, good-tasting, and predictable. That's why we favor glucose tablets. Most of the more convenient ones are imported: Dextrosols (from England) and Dextro-Energens (from Germany). From the United States you have B-D Glucose Tablets and the Orange Medical Company's Dextrotabs. All of these glucose tablets come in different flavors except B-Ds. Dextrosols, originally imported by Dr. Richard Bernstein will, he tells us, raise the blood sugar of a person weighing 120 to 150 pounds by approximately 15 milligrams per deciliter. Dextro-Energens raise blood sugar by 20 milligrams per deciliter and Dextrotabs by 8 milligrams per deciliter. The best way to find out exactly how much each of these tablets will raise *your* blood sugar is to test them on yourself. (Wait until your blood sugar is 100 or below; then eat one and retest in fifteen minutes.) If you know how many to eat for an insulin reaction, you won't make the classic mistake of overcompensating and sending yourself from 50 to 250. (This is called anxiety eating, and that term describes the phenomenon perfectly.)

If you get to the point where you are too far gone to chew but are conscious and able to swallow, the suggested treatment is one of the jels that can be absorbed in the mouth. These are Glutose (in a plastic container), Insta-Glucose (in a squeeze tube), and Monoject Insulin Reaction Gel (foil-wrapped pouch). A less expensive way to go is to pick up a few tubes of cake decorating icing in any supermarket.

Our final word: If you take insulin, live like a Boy Scout. Be prepared.

I've been told I should keep a supply of glucagon on hand. What is glucagon, and how is it used?

Glucagon is a hormone that's injected in the same way as insulin, only it has the opposite effect. It raises blood sugar. It's used to resuscitate diabetics who are unconscious because of low blood sugar.

Even if you never use it, glucagon is a nice security blanket. Just be sure whoever might be giving you an injection of glucagon knows where you keep it and how to administer it. And caution your family members or friends that if you're in insulin shock and unconscious, they should inject glucagon rather than trying to force liquid or food down your throat. An unconscious person cannot swallow and may choke to death.

Glucagon is available by prescription only. (This has never made sense to us, since insulin *isn't* a prescription medication and it's essential to have a supply of glucagon on hand if you take insulin.) It comes in two forms: Glucagon for Injection USP, which means you need a one-cubic-centimeter syringe and have to mix it before injection, and Glucagon Emergency Kit, which is preferable because the syringe is supplied and already filled with diluting solution. Many pharmacies do not regularly carry glucagon. When you find one that does or will order it for you, check the expiration date of glucagon before purchase. Glucagon for Injection USP is good for five years; the kit expires in one year. Prices can be very high, so comparison shop. (The kit is now around twenty-five dollars.)

I'm afraid of having an insulin reaction when I'm asleep and never waking up. Can this happen?

This is so rare that we've heard of it happening only twice. One time it was a diabetic who went to bed drunk and wound up literally dead drunk. What happened was the alcohol suppressed the body's method of spontaneous recovery. Normally, the liver converts some of its stored starch to glucose, and that saves you. The moral of this story is to always go to bed sober.

The other instance was reported to us by the sister of a young man who died. She said he was so obsessively compulsive about never having a slightly elevated blood sugar that he always played it too close. One night he went to bed and didn't wake up. His sister found his blood-sugar record book and discovered that his before-bed blood sugar was 70. Obviously, he needed a snack before bed and either didn't have one or had too little. The moral of this story is not to be a fanatic about your blood-sugar control.

There is an instrument that can give you more peace of mind at night. It's called the Sleep Sentry. It measures two symptoms of low blood sugar—a drop in temperature, and perspiration on the skin. When either of these occurs, the Sleep Sentry beeps you awake so you can do something about it. The problem is that it doesn't work for everyone, since not everyone has these symptoms (June is one who doesn't), and it sometimes gives false alarms. But those for whom it *does* work consider it a security blanket and a sleep and sanity preserver.

What is diabetic coma?

A diabetic coma occurs when your blood sugar is extremely high—perhaps over 1,000. You have diabetic ketoacidosis. Your sodium-bicarbonate and carbon-dioxide levels are low. You are dehydrated. Oddly enough, you don't have to be unconscious to be in diabetic coma. Only 15 percent of those in diabetic coma are.

To define it more bluntly, diabetic coma is what out-of-control diabetics die of. Death from diabetic coma has been totally preventable since the discovery of insulin in 1921.

To avoid getting yourself into this dangerous state:

■ Do your best to always keep your diabetes under control.

■ Never neglect testing your blood sugar. If it's high, test for ketones, too. If there are ketones, call your doctor.

- If you are insulin-dependent, never neglect taking your injection.

- Whenever you are ill, check with your doctor to see if you need to take more insulin.

Diabetic coma approaches slowly. The symptoms are thirst, frequent urination, fever, drowsiness, rapid breathing, vomiting or nausea, and finally unconsciousness. The treatment for keto-acidosis is regular insulin.

Can I get a driver's license if I take insulin?

Definitely yes. We don't know the regulations in all states, be-cause they're all somewhat different, but we do know that the California Department of Motor Vehicles has liberal rules. Dia-betics don't even have to reveal that they have diabetes unless they're subject to periods of unconsciousness.

Is it all right to drive a car alone on long trips?

Of course. You must, however, always carefully monitor your blood sugar. On *any* trip, short or long, never start out before checking your blood sugar and making sure it is normal or some-what above normal. This should be a strict, no-exceptions-made personal law. We've heard of too many tragedies involving Sugar-Free clients not to be fervent advocates of this policy. This is one of June's most inflexible rules, and she was lucky enough to learn it through other people's experience. Driving is dangerous enough without augmenting the risk with a fuzzy mind and an ill-coordinated body,

It goes without saying that you should have glucose tablets and snacks in the car with you. If you're on a long trip, stop at regular intervals (say, every hour) and test your blood sugar. Then you can snack enough to avoid low blood sugar. And if you take NPH or any other intermediate or long-acting insulin that programs you into certain eating hours, you should stop and eat when mealtime strikes. If you know there's a dearth of restaurants on the route or you're particular about what you eat, it's better to take along a picnic meal than to risk having to delay your meal or stoke up on snacks.

Is is okay to exercise alone if you take insulin?

It's always better to have a companion for safety's sake, as well as for company. You especially shouldn't do anything potentially hazardous like skiing or swimming alone.

Still, there isn't always somebody around, and a diabetic does always need exercise. There's no reason you can't take a walk or jog or ride your bicycle or play a round of golf by yourself. Just be sure you never leave the house without glucose tablets and enough snacks to see you through. *Enough* is the word here. Take along a lot more than you think you can possibly need. Then you'll never have to curtail your fun. Choose snacks that are good and, preferably, good for you, such as small packages of raisins or dried prunes, Fi-Bars, fruit leathers, trail mix, fruit-juice-sweetened cookies, peanut butter and crackers, and the like.

For
Non-Insulin-Dependent
Diabetics (Type II)

· ·

We recently spoke to the fourth-year medical students at the University of Southern California, after which we had the opportunity to chat with one of the professors there, Maureen Strohm, M.D. She had what we considered a brilliant and obvious theory. (We find that brilliant theories often seem obvious once the originators point them out.)

It is Dr. Strohm's theory that with most overweight Type II diabetics, diabetes is a symptom. The real disease is overweight, and that's what should be treated. Her theory is reinforced by the National Institutes of Health panel's statement that "overweight of any degree is a disease. Obesity is a killer." (*Obesity* is defined as 20 percent or more over ideal body weight.)

We then evolved the theory that Type II diabetes is really a lifestyle disease. When we checked this out with Dr. Lois Jovanovic-Peterson, she said this was true in the case of those

161

who are diabetic as a complication of obesity. Lean Type II's are victims of chance and heredity.

But 80 percent of Type II's *are* overweight, and this poses insidious treatment problems. If you treat the diabetes, giving more and more blood-sugar-lowering pills or injecting more and more insulin to bring blood sugar down, the person is likely to eat as much or more and gain weight (insulin is a potent fat-building hormone). With the weight gain, insulin resistance will increase and the symptom of diabetes will become more and more severe.

On the other hand, if the disease of overweight is effectively treated and the weight goes down, the symptom of diabetes may well disappear, giving you normal blood sugar without pills and without insulin. Mind you, the diabetes will still be there waiting in the wings. It will come onstage again if your weight goes up, but as long as you keep the disease of overweight in control, and as long as no other risk factor develops, diabetes won't play a major part in your life.

So if you're an overweight diabetic, the most important change you can make is to lose those extra pounds and lose them forever. Overweight isn't, after all, a chronic and incurable disease. You can treat it, you can cure it, and you can restore yourself to health.

We realize this is much easier said than done. In some ways it's easier to control diabetes with insulin or a pill than it is to control your weight. As Dr. Jovanovic-Peterson points out in *The Diabetic Woman*, most Type II women became obese from an eating disorder to begin with. Therefore, help with the disorder through a hospital program and/or a support group such as Overeaters Anonymous may be the first step to take. But even without an eating disorder, Type II's should pay particular attention to the information in earlier sections of this book on diet and exercise.

Ironically, if you have a fear of needles, it might be of help. Sometimes just the idea that you'll have to take insulin is enough to inspire the dramatic weight loss needed. But, as always, we prefer positive motivation. Think how much better you'll feel, how much better you'll look, and how much longer you'll live without those excess pounds—and without that bothersome symptom known as diabetes.

What does it mean to be told you're a "borderline" diabetic?

It means the person who told you that has a very loose grasp on what diabetes is all about. There is no such thing as "borderline" diabetes. The term has been outmoded since 1979, when the National Diabetes Data Group came up with the Type I and Type II classifications of diabetes for insulin-dependent and non-insulin-dependent diabetes. Before that time Type I was called juvenile-onset, and Type II maturity-onset. Since age of onset of diabetes does not determine the type of diabetes (see page 166 about Type II children), these terms are considered misleading and inaccurate.

The new classification system also wiped out such fuzzy and often misunderstood terms as "chemical diabetes," subclinical diabetes," "asymptomatic diabetes," and "latent diabetes." All of these terms were replaced with "impaired glucose tolerance."

In a report published in the journal *Diabetes*, it was pointed out that impaired glucose tolerance is not diabetes and the use of the label "diabetes" for people with "marginal" blood levels "can invoke social, psychological, and economic sanctions that are unjustified in the light of the lack of severity of their glucose intolerance." (Translation: These people shouldn't be denied jobs that are forbidden to diabetics.)

The glucose-tolerance-test graph (Figure 1) shows the difference in glucose levels among a nondiabetic, a person with impaired glucose tolerance, and a diabetic.

As *Diabetes Forecast* points out, "while some people whose blood-glucose levels are somewhat elevated *do* develop diabetes, many people subsequently have normal tests and continue to test 'normal' indefinitely."

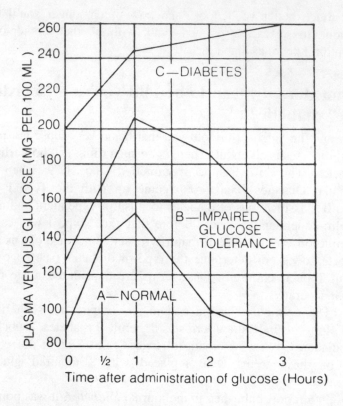

FIGURE 1. The three people represented on this graph each had 100 grams of glucose administered by mouth. One person (A-Normal) is nondiabetic. One person (B-Normal) has impaired glucose tolerance. And the other person (C-DM) is diabetic, either insulin-dependent or non-insulin-dependent. You can see that the nondiabetic's body has removed most of the glucose from circulation within two hours. In the diabetic, whose glucose levels were already too high, the glucose level shot even higher than at first, and three hours later the levels had not yet begun to drop. The person with impaired glucose tolerance has a curve similar to that of the nondiabetic, except that it is somewhat higher. Also, at the end of two hours this person's glucose level had dropped only slightly, whereas the nondiabetic's blood-glucose level had returned to normal. *(Courtesy of Gerald R. Cooper, M.D., Ph.D.,* Diabetes Forecast, *March–April 1980, p. 39. Copyright 1980 by the American Diabetes Association. Reprinted from* Diabetes Forecast *with permission.)*

Our personal opinion is that if you have impaired glucose tolerance you should follow the diabetic lifestyle just to be on the safe side. But then we feel that *everybody* should follow the diabetic lifestyle.

I've heard that Type II diabetes isn't as serious as Type I diabetes. Is this true?

It's about as true as saying that if you forget about diabetes it will go away. We wish it were true, because then instead of 12 million diabetics in the United States there would be only 1 million. And we wish it were true for your sake, if you are a Type II, because that would mean you could relax and put your condition in the same category as a food allergy or a case of eczema.

No, it's not true. Type II diabetes is just as serious as Type I, and, like Type I, it will, if ignored or neglected, eventually cause the same serious health problems. The only difference is that the pattern of the development of these problems and their types may be somewhat different. Uncontrolled Type II diabetes leads most often to heart disease, strokes, high blood pressure, and foot problems, while uncontrolled Type I diabetes is more likely to create eye, kidney, and nerve damage (in scientific terms, retinopathy, nephropathy, and neuropathy, respectively). Of course, Type II's can develop any of those complications also. In fact, Priscilla Hollander, M.D., writing in *Learning to Live Well with Diabetes*, says, "Neuropathy seems to appear earlier in people with Type II diabetes. In fact, it may be the first sign that a person has Type II diabetes."

A more positive piece of information is that these threats to your health do not develop fast. It takes eight or ten or even fifteen years for the body gradually to succumb to them. You do have to consider, however, that if you had high blood sugar several years before you were diagnosed diabetic, some damage could have been done even before you were aware of your diabetes. This would explain why the development of neuropathy might be the first clue to your doctor that you have developed diabetes. As with many other diseases, the sooner you discover you have diabetes, the better off you are, because you can start normalizing your blood sugar and thereby prevent or reverse complications.

If you put two and two together you'll notice that the leading complications of Type II diabetes are the same as those problems that tend to develop as you move into your more advanced years. In other word, Type II diabetes and aging both move you in the direction of heart disease, strokes, high blood pressure, and foot problems, especially if your lifestyle has been and continues to be unhealthy (very little exercise, high-fat diet, stress, smoking, etc.) and your family has a history of these diseases. Therefore, if you're already in your fifties or sixties, the threat of dying of heart disease or stroke is now escalated because you have developed diabetes as an additional risk factor. All the more reason to play it safe and follow the lifestyle of the great numbers of active, health-conscious seniors we now have in this country.

Can children have Type II diabetes?

Maybe. (How's that for an equivocal answer?) Richard Guthrie, M.D., of the Diabetes Treatment Center at St. Joseph's Medical Center in Wichita, Kansas, and Diana Guthrie, R.N., Ph.D., of the University of Kansas School of Medicine in Wichita, tell us:

> Overweight children with high blood-sugar levels are brought to our attention by referral from other physicians or parents who are concerned about the weight problem in the child. When we do a glucose-tolerance test on them, we also analyze for insulin values. These particular children, who usually have high glucose levels as well as high insulin values, return to normal laboratory values in most cases once weight loss has been achieved. We have not followed them to find out about complications, but we have seen

some children in this descriptive category become Type II diabetics. The main treatment, of course, is increasing the activity
level with the ultimate goal of decreasing the weight. Usually, the
children are not on restricted caloric intake, but we work very
strongly with maintaining the caloric intake and increasing the
activity level.

Since I don't take insulin, do I have to do all that blood-sugar testing?

Absolutely. All diabetics who want to keep normal blood-sugar
levels, and that should be your goal, have to test their blood sugar
to assure themselves that they are staying on track. No way out.
Well, there is an illusory way out. You may have been put on old-
fashioned urine-sugar testing instead of blood-sugar testing and
led to believe that if there is no sugar in your urine, your blood
sugar is okay. Supposedly, no sugar in the urine means you are
staying under 180—the normal renal threshold, as it is called. It
is the normal level at which sugar moves into the urine in a
desperate attempt to keep you out of what Dr. Peter Forsham
calls "glucotoxicity" (sugars high enough to poison your
system).

But this is the rub: since most people are older when diagnosed and the renal threshold goes up with age, finding no sugar
in your urine may simply mean that your renal threshold has
edged up. But your blood sugar might still be dangerously high.
This is common with older Type II's who may have been introduced to urine testing years ago when it was the only test you
could take.

For example, we talked to the daughter of a diabetic woman
who, according to her daughter, "*loves* to eat, especially at big
family gatherings." The mother would take her urine test, it
would show that she wasn't spilling sugar, and so, presuming her
blood sugar to be normal, she'd sit down happily and, as her
daughter put it, "have a feast."

The woman wound up in the hospital with dangerous ketoacidosis. She'd been running extremely high blood sugar, but it had never shown up in her urine because of her high renal threshold.

This woman is now testing her blood sugar regularly at home. She doesn't have many feasts these days, but she's going to be around for a lot more regular meals than she would have been had she continued to dwell in a diabetic's fool's paradise with her urine tests.

Another insidious aspect about being casual with your self-care and testing is that if you run around too long with elevated blood sugar, those diabetes complications we described on pages 16–18 can start slowly and quietly developing. You may never even know what is going on until the damage is done. We're not fear mongers, and we don't like to threaten you with the problems diabetics are heir to, but in our experience many non-insulin-dependent diabetics don't get the point about the seriousness of diabetes the way insulin takers do.

Remember that even if you don't take insulin, you have to be as careful as any other diabetic. Actually, non-insulin takers are the most likely candidates for arrival at the hospital with diabetes-related complications or, as diabetes nurse specialist Diana Guthrie warns, "to have to have part of a leg removed," because they're the ones most likely to ignore their diabetes until it screams for attention.

My doctor has prescribed pills to help me control my blood-sugar levels. What are these, and are they safe?

They are oral drugs that help lower blood sugar in some Type II diabetics. They are not oral insulin, as some people think. (Insulin cannot effectively be taken orally, as it is a protein and is digested.) These drugs can increase the amount of insulin your pancreas is producing, and they seem to influence the way insulin acts to lower blood sugar.

These oral hypoglycemics, as the doctors call them, all belong to one class of drugs, the sulfonylureas. The first generation of sulfonylureas (known generically as tolbutamide, chlorpropamide acetohexamide, and tolazamide) carry an FDA warning about their causing an increased risk of heart attack (just what you don't need). The second generation of oral hypoglycemics (generically called glyburide and glipizide), which came into use in the United States in 1984, are much more potent and are considered safer in that they cause fewer side effects because the dosage is small and they do not interact with other drugs. Table 4 shows the entire choice of sulfonylurea drugs now available.

Generic Name	Trade Name	Available Dosage Strengths, Tablets (mg)	Maximum Dosage (gm/day)	Duration Action (hours)
FIRST GENERATION				
Tolbutamide	Orinase	250–500	2.0–3.0	6–12
Chlorpropamide	Diabinase	100–250	0.5	up to 600
Acetohexamide	Dymelor	250–500	1.5	12–24
Tolazamide	Tolinase	100–250–500	1.5	10–16
SECOND GENERATION				
Glyburide	Micronase[R]	1.25–2.5 to 5	20 mg	18–30
Glyburide	Diabeta[R]	1.25–2.5 to 5	20 mg	18–30
Glipizide	Glucotrol[R]	5 to 10	40 mg	14–20

TABLE 4. Oral hypoglycemics.

Oral drug therapy is a next-to-the-last-resort treatment for Type II diabetes. The first line of defense is diet and exercise. Then if blood sugars do not retreat, the person is a candidate for some kind of pill. If pills alone don't cause improvement, you can take advantage of a new technique being tried: combining pills with one shot of insulin a day, usually a small amount of intermediate-acting NPH at bedtime. The disadvantage here is that the insulin may increase obesity.

If you are using oral drugs, you do need to monitor your blood sugar on a regular basis. Since the advent of the newer, stronger oral drugs, you must watch particularly for low blood sugar. The second-generation drugs are likely to cause more hypoglycemia, because they are more effective. If you use one of them, eat your meals regularly and check your blood sugar when you exercise or when you have symptoms of hypoglycemia: sweating, shaking, dizziness, slurred speech, blurred vision, hunger, irritability, nausea, or confusion.

You also need to check your blood sugar, because many people have what is known as "secondary failure" on their oral drug. Sixty percent of the people who initially got good results with first-generation pills, which have been used in the United States for thirty-two years, failed on them after six years. The hope is that this experience won't be repeated with the second-generation drugs.

Obviously, if you fail on the pills the next step is insulin.

How am I able to lose weight quickly, easily, and permanently?

You can't. But then you already knew that, didn't you? If it were possible to lose weight quickly, easily, and permanently, you wouldn't have a weight problem and neither would the 40 percent of the people over forty in the United States who are classified as overweight.

No, weight loss—if it is accomplished at all—comes slowly and with difficulty, and you're always at risk of putting the weight back on again.

But that doesn't mean you can't do it. You can. After all, you have that great motivator—diabetes. You want to lose weight to keep your diabetes under control and possibly to stay off insulin. That should give you a lot more incentive than just reasons of general good health or vanity. (But don't discount vanity as a motivator for losing weight. The desire to look good is right up there with the desire to feel good. Snap up any reason you can to make yourself truly want to work at losing weight.)

Once the desire is there, though, how do you go about doing it? There are plenty of people out there who want to help you—usually for a price. That's where you have to be careful. The faster the weight comes off using some kind of strange fad diet or program, the more likely it is to come back again. A crash diet invariably crashes. It is very bad for your health to bounce back and forth from weight loss to weight gain to weight loss and so on.

Magazines that have to fill their pages up with something frequently fill them with ideas for losing weight that run from the sublime ("fall in love") to the ridiculous ("chew each mouthful of food thirty-two times"). But strangely enough, some of these ideas have a kernel of truth in them, and if you can incorporate some of them into a sensible, sound weight-loss program, why not do it?

Falling in love is a great idea. An intense emotional experience could take your mind off food and instill you with the desire to be attractive to the loved one. (But it's probably even harder to run out and find someone to fall in love with than to lose weight in a more conventional albeit more boring way.)

Chewing your food thirty-two times is actually based on a theory by Horace Fletcher, a nineteenth-century nutritionist who believed you should chew food that number of times for the logical reason that we have thirty-two teeth. You hardly need to chew *that* much, but chewing food thoroughly rather than gulping it down slows the eating process and gives your body a better chance of signaling to you that you're no longer hungry.

To hark back to the first section of this book, if you can make yourself happy, that can help you lose weight. Contrary to the old idea that fat people are happy, it's often unhappiness that sends people running to the refrigerator for solace.

There are other, easier-to-achieve techniques that can also help. For example, when you eat, do nothing but eat. You can engage in some delightful dinner-table conversation, but don't read or watch television, because if you're not paying attention to your food, you tend to just unconsciously shovel it in. On top of that you don't enjoy it very much, and food should be pleasurable. We've noticed that the better tasting and more enjoyable food is, the sooner you feel fully satisfied with a meal, so you tend to eat less.

Another valid tip is to eat in only one place in the house—in your dining room or at your kitchen table. That way you don't wander around snacking all the time. (Snacks are often what do a weight-loss program in.)

Another sound suggestion is to write down everything you eat—and we do mean everything, right down to the breath mint you have after lunch. Seeing in black and white what you've eaten and the number of calories it contains can vividly show you where you're going wrong and where those unwanted pounds are coming from. It also gets pretty tedious writing all that stuff down, so conceivably you'll start deciding to skip the snack to avoid having to get out your notebook and record it. Actually, a University of Pittsburgh School of Medicine study showed that Type II diabetics on a weight-loss program who meticulously recorded what they ate lost an average of thirty-seven pounds, whereas those who wrote in a haphazard and irregular way lost an average of only ten pounds. Two good record books can help you keep track of your food and exercise: the *Lifestyle Record Book* (HCF Nutrition Research Foundation, Box 22124, Lexington, Kentucky 40522) and *Dietchecker* (Lifestyle Systems, Box 9983, San Diego, California 92109-0340).

The Pittsburgh-study diabetics also recorded their daily exercise, for, indeed, that is the other half of a sensible and effective weight-loss program. It may even be two-thirds or three-quarters of the program. It's that important. Weight lost with a combination of diet and exercise comes off faster and is much more likely to stay off than weight taken off by diet alone. That makes sense because weight loss is brought about by burning more calories than you consume—and exercise burns calories.

Something else burns calories: your metabolism. Your physical and mental processes burn calories even while you're sitting still or asleep. Some people have rapid rates of metabolism—the lucky devils. These are the people who can stuff down mountains of anything they want to eat and remain as skinny as a broom handle. Others have a slow metabolism, and even when they eat very lightly they puff up like a vacuum-cleaner bag.

In the past, people who claimed it was their metabolism that caused them to be overweight were winked at behind their backs by those accusing them of being secret stuffers. Now studies are revealing that many of them were telling the truth. Their low metabolic rate was what frustrated their attempts at weight loss.

If you're one of these slow metabolizers, that doesn't mean you should just throw up your hands and feel doomed to being overweight. You can rev up your metabolism—by exercise. That's the whole principle behind many effective weight-loss theories, including Covert Bailey's *Fit or Fat* series of books and Martin Katahn's *Beyond Diet*. Exercise has the additional advantage of suppressing your appetite. One of our nutritional heroes, Dr. Jean Mayer, summed up the situation: "You have three choices: you can exercise more, you can always feel hungry, or you can be fat." It's obvious which is the best choice.

Speaking of choices, when selecting foods, little things can make a big difference. Just as the Glycemic Index is a good guide to choosing the foods that raise your blood sugar slower and less, two guides to keep in mind for reducing are *fiber* and *fat*. Go for the foods that are higher in fiber. They fill you up better while giving you fewer calories. And run from the foods that are higher in fat. Fat has over twice the calories of carbohydrates and proteins. Some people have been able to peel off pounds by the simple expedient of avoiding fats. This is one of the cornerstones of the Pritikin weight-loss program.

Incidentally, Pritikin is one of the many weight-loss programs that entice you with advertising of their formidable benefits. And a number of these *are* effective and worth looking into. When you're looking into them, though, you should take into consideration their cost and exactly what the diet involves that they require you to follow. Check out the former with your bank account and the latter with your physician or dietitian to see if it's appropriate for your diabetes.

Also, some weight-loss support groups can be very effective, as long as they are truly supportive and don't make a ritual of ridiculing people who haven't reached their week's goal for weight loss. One of our nondiabetic employees achieved great and long-lasting success with Overeaters Anonymous. If you do find a compatible group, it can do a lot to inspire you. Losing weight is like dying; it's something you ultimately have to do alone, but it's nice to have someone there to hold your hand while it's happening.

Are those liquid diets good for diabetic weight-loss programs?

They are more for people who fall into the obese rather than the overweight category. The renowned Mayo Clinic recommends such plans only for people who are at least fifty pounds overweight or 30 percent heavier than what would be considered their ideal weight. These diets should be undertaken only under the advice and careful guidance of a physician. This holds true for anybody—but especially for a diabetic.

For Family
and Friends

. . . .

They say that one person in four is touched by diabetes. That is to say, you have it, you eventually will have it, or you are a family member or close friend of someone who has it. Since you're reading this section, you probably fall into one of the two latter categories. And you have your problems, too.

June, in her more mellow moments, allows that she thinks diabetes is sometimes harder on family members and friends of diabetics than on the diabetics themselves. She may be right, especially when it comes to the parents of diabetic children. For many of them their guilt feelings, anguish, and constant worry are exquisite torture. Parents often lie awake fretting through the night while in the next room their diabetic child sleeps—appropriately enough—like a baby.

Some adult diabetics manage to lay all the responsibility for their care on a spouse. In these cases it's usually—but certainly not always—the wife of a diabetic who learns the diabetic diet, prepares it, and tries to see to it that her husband sticks to it while he remains aloof and unconcerned. On the other hand, we had a husband drop by a SugarFree Center who did the blood-sugar testing for his diabetic wife. He took the blood sample,

175

read it, recorded the results—in short, handled everything—because she refused to have anything to do with it.

Friends of diabetics sometimes encounter the opposite situation. The diabetic doesn't want to impose his or her problem on someone else and so will hardly talk about it, let alone clue in the friend on how to help on a day-to-day basis or even in time of emergency.

It's never easy. In a sense your family members and friends are like insulin-taking diabetics who walk a tightrope between high and low blood sugar. Only the tightrope you walk is between not doing enough and doing too much, between being oblivious to a diabetic's problems and being concerned to the point of driving the diabetic—and yourself—crazy.

In this section we'll try to help you with your delicate and nerve-wracking balancing act and show you that although you're touched by diabetes, you don't have to be pushed around, pummeled, and knocked out by it.

By the way, it's a good idea for you to read *all* the questions in this section, even the ones that on the surface don't appear to apply to you. You may find just the help you need buried in a seemingly unrelated situation.

Will diabetes make changes in our family life?

Only about as many changes as moving a hippopotamus into the living room. Each looms large on the scene, can't be ignored, has to be worked around, demands a great deal of time and trouble and care; and you never stop wishing that someone would take the damned thing away.

But strangely enough, you can get used to anything, be it hippopotamus or diabetes. Eventually when people express shock and concern—"Oh, you have a hippopotamus in your living room!" (or "Oh, your child, husband, or wife has diabetes!") "How terrible!"—you're surprised they even mention it as an oddity or a problem. It's just what *is*, a part of your life—and you're living with it.

How do I help the diabetic in my life?

Learn. Learn all you can about diabetes. Become a walking encyclopedia of diabetes lore so you can be an intelligent and informed as well as a caring partner. Notice we say *partner*. Don't do it all. Don't try to take over. Don't make the diabetic—child or adult—totally dependent on you. That's not an act of kindness. Diabetics have to be responsible for themselves. After all, you can't be around every minute—and even if you can you shouldn't be.

It's especially important for you to attend diabetes education classes and diabetes-association meetings with the diabetic. Not only does this give emotional support, but two sets of eyes and ears absorbing the information make the program twice as effective.

If you have a diabetic child, we especially recommend that you join the Juvenile Diabetes Foundation International (see Reference Section: Directory of Organizations). Their primary goal is the worthy one of raising funds to finance research toward a cure for diabetes. But membership in this organization has the additional value of putting you in touch with other parents of diabetics with whom you can share problems and—more important—solutions.

Another way to learn about diabetes is somewhat unusual, but if you're up to doing it, it will increase your understanding of diabetes tremendously and also help you develop empathy for the diabetic. Empathy is better than sympathy. Sympathy is feeling sorry for people; empathy is feeling how they feel, almost getting inside their skin.

Here's the way: you live exactly as a diabetic lives for a period of time. This idea was developed at the Diabetic Unit of the Queen Elizabeth II Medical Center in Western Australia, where they believed that the staff who treated diabetics needed to know what their patients' lives were really like. Volunteers for the experiment were required to take injections, using a saline solution instead of insulin, test their blood, eat the diabetic diet, including snacks at the proper time, etc. These educators had to "be diabetic" for only a week, but some of them couldn't last even that long. The only one who was really successful at it just gave up her social life entirely and stayed at home catering to her diabetes. That, of course, isn't the way to do it. You're supposed to lead a normal life. After all, that's the goal for diabetics, and that's what everyone else is always telling them they can do.

As Dr. Martyn Sulway, the physician in charge of the program, put it, "They found out having diabetes isn't a piece of cake." (Australian pronunciation: "pace of kaike.")

Barbara, even though she thought she knew all she needed to about the diabetic life, decided to try the experiment, because she'd been haranguing diabetics for years about what they ought to do yet had no firsthand experience. She did it, not for a week but for a month. It was a relevation.

Although she'd always bragged about eating the diabetes diet, she discovered that she hadn't been nearly as meticulous about it as a diabetic needs to be. For example, she hadn't always turned down *every* dessert. Also, she hadn't had to be continually worrying about keeping the inexorable snack on hand for an emergency, *and*—this irritated her the most—she hadn't had to eat when she wasn't hungry.

She took twice-daily blood sugars (and to her surprise discovered that she may have a twinge of reactive hypoglycemia). She took three injections a day. In order to have a little health hype out of it, she shot vitamin B_{12} instead of saline solution. Strangely enough, the injections weren't as bad as expected. At first they were an interesting novelty, but before long they became just a bore. Occasionally and for no apparent reason the shots hurt, but most of the time they were relatively painless.

She even managed to get the flu (not deliberately) and decided that if she really had been a diabetic she would have wound up in the hospital because her diabetes-care program fell totally to pieces. This really brought home how important it is for a diabetic to avoid getting the minor diseases that go around every year.

Barbara also developed a greater tolerance for the foibles and peccadillos of diabetics. She has always been aghast at reports that some teenagers (and even one diabetic celebrity) shoot through their clothes when out in restaurants. But one night during the first week of the experiment she was dining out with friends and suddenly realized halfway through the meal that she'd forgotten to take her "insulin." So *zap!*—right through the old corduroy pants and into the leg.

One of the worst features of "having diabetes," Barbara found, was having to keep your mind cluttered with it every minute. As June says, it's as if you're always playing an intricate chess game on top of whatever else you're doing.

The *truly* worst feature of diabetes—the worry about hypoglycemia and long-term complications—can't be duplicated in a nondiabetic. Still, you can learn an amazing amount.

Why should I follow the diabetic diet and exercise plan?

It will help keep the diabetic doing it. But that's not the main reason. The main reason is that it will maintain your own good health. There's nothing peculiar about the diabetic lifestyle. It's what we all should be doing. If you read the recommendations for good health from the Department of Agriculture and Department of Health and Human Services, or the American Heart Association, you'll see they're nothing more than the well-balanced meals with fresh fruits and vegetables, whole grains, no concentrated sweets, and reduced fats recommended for diabetics. The diabetes exercise program, too—regular amounts of aerobic exercise—is exactly what everyone should be doing, according to all fitness experts.

Actually, having a diabetic in your life or home is a tremendous boon. It wakes the entire family up to the best way of living and gives them an incentive for doing it.

It's particularly valuable when there are nondiabetic children in the family. If a sister or brother or parent has diabetes and the house is therefore bereft of junk food, they're going to develop healthy eating habits that will stay with them all through life.

Then, too, if any of the nondiabetics have the genetic gun loaded with a diabetic tendency, leading the diabetic lifestyle may well keep the trigger from ever being pulled.

And here's what may be the most effective inducement: If you have a diabetic spouse and he or she follows the diet and exercise program and you don't, you won't be able to measure up to your youthfully lean and vital counterpart. This can be bad for the dynamics of the marriage, to say nothing of your ego.

We feel compelled to warn you, however, of a built-in hazard when you're a nondiabetic in the company of a diabetic. That hazard is the old slip twixt the cup (and the fork and the spoon) and the lip. In other words, although you know better, you are constantly tempted to eat for two, and, alas, you often succumb to that temptation.

Here's how it works. The well-behaved diabetic is eye-measuring his or her food at a meal and eating right on the diet. You're doing pretty much the same, or maybe you're eating a *little* more, because after all you don't have to be all that careful with your measurements.

Then it turns out there are leftovers. They'll never be so tasty again. In fact, it would be foolish to try to keep them. And you don't want to waste all that good food. Think of the starving people around the world. So . . . down the hatch.

A few hours pass, and if the diabetic takes insulin it's time for a snack because he or she has to have small amounts of food at regular intervals to feed the insulin. As long as the diabetic is munching you figure you might as well be companionable and munch along. Your snack, which, again, doesn't have to be so carefully measured, goes down the hatch.

Dining out is even more tempting and hazardous. Perhaps there's a bottle of wine and the diabetic permits him- or herself one three-ounce glass. Somebody has to drink the rest. It cost a lot of money. You can't send it back, and they don't have doggie bags for liquids. Down the hatch.

Maybe there's a really fantastic dessert selection and the dessert comes with the meal. The diabetic prudently says no. Two desserts go down the hatch.

When you and the diabetic are at a friend's home for dinner, your eating for two becomes almost a social necessity. The hostess has worked so very hard on hors d'oeuvres and exotic concoctions—especially exotic dessert concoctions—that she's going to be wounded right down to the bottom of her saucepan if *someone* doesn't lap up with gusto everything in sight and ask for more. The diabetic can't. It's up to you. Down the hatch.

If this keeps up, before too long that hatch of yours is going to be attached to a tub, a tub that is in imminent danger of sinking. This is especially true if the diabetic in your life is a relative, such as a sister or brother, with whom you share the same heredity. In this case, with your eating for two you could chomp your way into Diabetesland.

You have been warned. If you don't want that long and healthy life insurance policy the diabetic has provided for you canceled, you have to pay the premium. That premium is to exert the same self-control as the diabetic and eat for only one. Then close down the hatch.

Should I marry a diabetic?

That, like the decision to marry at all, has ultimately to be your own decision, as you undoubtedly well know. The probable reason for asking this is that you're concerned about the problems your potential mate's diabetes might cause in the future.

It's wise to think about these possible problems now rather than later. As diabetes teaching nurse Diane Victor said to a young man who was complaining about some aspect of his wife's diabetes and shirking his responsibility for helping to deal with it, "Look, you knew she was diabetic when you married her. You signed on for the duration. Shape up."

Diabetes is never problem free, as we've made clear in this book and as you have probably already personally observed if you have a close relationship with a diabetic. Diabetes care takes time, time you would prefer to spend on more entertaining activities. Diabetes care takes money, money you would prefer to spend on other things. Diabetes can make having children more difficult, hazardous, and—again—expensive. And diabetes, if not cared for properly and controlled, can eventually cause debilitating complications and an earlier death.

But all of this doesn't mean you should give back (or take back) the engagement ring. Marriage is full of risks. You could marry a flawless specimen bearing a doctor's certificate of perfect health and the day after your wedding he or she or even *you* could get in an accident that paralyzed everything south of the earlobes. We have a friend whose apparently healthy wife developed multiple sclerosis in the first year they were married.

There are no guarantees in life. When you get married, the old "for better or for worse; in sickness and in health" still holds true. Realistically considered, diabetes, if well controlled, is one of the lesser worses and healthier sicknesses, and knowing about it in advance gives you a chance to learn and prepare and adjust.

Of course, it is possible for diabetes to destroy a marriage. Some marriages are so tenuous that they can't survive any adversity. In such cases, if it hadn't been diabetes that caused the breakup, something else would have.

Diabetes can also strengthen marriages. When one partner develops a potentially life-threatening condition, this makes the other realize how important the previously taken-for-granted person really is. Working together to control diabetes can, in fact, bring a new closeness. We heard of a long-married couple whose children had grown and who had gradually become so consumed by their individual interest that they hardly had anything left in common. Each was running on a separate track. When the wife was diagnosed diabetic, the tracks merged as they headed toward the same goal.

In the final analysis we believe that love conquers all. By this we don't mean the short-lived romantic love that turns your mind to irrational (but delicious) mush. No, we're referring to the enduring, day-to-day-growing love that comes from living through and living with problems together and helping each other play out whatever hands you may be dealt, trying to turn the game into a winning one.

Does a diabetic child disrupt a family?

A diabetic child can disrupt it or can merely change it, in some ways for the better. Disruptions occur when the parents are filled with guilt, anger, or both. We heard of a husband who blamed his wife for the child's diabetes and threatened to divorce her "if anything happens to that kid." Obviously, he hadn't heard of the theory of the cause of Type I diabetes being a virus, just as the cause of the measles or mumps is a virus.

Parents fraught with guilt can coddle and overindulge a diabetic child. This not only creates resentment and feelings of being unloved in any other children in the family but can be ruinous for the diabetic child as well. Diabetes can become for the child an excuse for dependence and manipulation of other family members instead of a stepping-stone to strength.

On the other hand, psychologist Barbara Goldberg, writing in *Diabetes Forecast*, emphasized that every family of a diabetic child that she talked to "mentioned that, in spite of, or perhaps because of, the illness, there was a special protectiveness, helpfulness, and a greater sense of family closeness."

This also holds true if one parent becomes diabetic. In American families these days we tend to be more than somewhat child centered. If a parent becomes diabetic and needs attention and care from the rest of the family, this develops in the children an increased responsibility and sensitivity to the needs of others.

In one family, the father, who had flexible business hours, spent much of his spare time chauffeuring the kids to their many and varied sporting activities and cheering them on from the sidelines. When he developed diabetes and had a need for exercise himself, the kids made it their business to see that dad got his jog every day and took turns accompanying him on it. New responsibilities. New closeness.

What can I do for my diabetic child?

There are many things you can do. You can help the child accept the disease and teach him or her how to take care of it. You can encourage diabetic children to achieve whatever they want to achieve in life despite diabetes. But there's one extremely important thing parents sometimes fail to do because they don't know it needs to be done—help diabetic children get rid of some of the terrible fears they carry around inside and suffer over and don't talk about.

Dr. Robert Rood, a San Fernando Valley diabetologist who works with children and adolescents, told a story about a child at a summer camp where he was serving as physician. This girl was a model camper, full of fun and very popular.

Dr. Rood, in checking out her blood tests, discovered that her one shot of insulin a day wasn't doing the job. (These were the old days when one shot a day was typical.) He decided to divide her insulin into two doses—morning and evening. This worked fine. Her blood sugar returned to normal. But *she* became very *ab*normal—sullen, negative, picking fights. When he took her aside to talk, she broke down and started crying. "I don't want to die," she said between sobs.

"Die?" said Dr. Rood. "Why are you talking about dying?"

"I know my diabetes was bad before when I had to take one

shot. *Now* it must be getting lots worse because I have to take two. I'm going to die. I know it."

Dr. Rood reassured her, of course, and she became her old self again, but he had learned something important. You never know what's going on in a child's head. You have to take the time to talk and explain. Be especially careful if there are any major changes in diabetes routines, lest the child interpret them as Dr. Rood's camper did.

Diabetic children also sometimes believe their diabetes is a punishment for "being bad." This gives them guilt feelings as well as fear if they're ever "bad" again something even worse will happen.

And don't overlook the hidden fears and guilts of the non-diabetic children in the family. Younger children can get the idea that when they reach the age when the older child got it, they'll get diabetes, too. Each day to them becomes like the tick of a time bomb.

Guilt feelings arise when nondiabetic children have harbored some quite normal sibling-rivalry evil thoughts, like "I wish Eddie would die," and lo, Eddie gets diabetes. They hold themselves responsible.

Parents must be aware of these dangers when the element of diabetes enters the family. Diabetes means there must be closer communication, more understanding, and more openness in the family. And that's all to the good.

If my diabetic child goes to a birthday party or trick-or-treating on Halloween, is it all right to break the diet just this once?

Think how many "just this once's" that would make in a year. Before long, just this once becomes an everyday occurrence and bad habits are established. Your child's health and maybe even life expectancy are diminished.

It's hard to see your child deprived when other kids are

loading up on goodies—maybe it's even harder on you than on the child—but diabetes is going to be there all his or her life. Now is when lifetime behavior patterns are established. You're *not* being kind when you let your child break his or her diet just this once.

One thing you can do on occasions when your child is being deprived is figure out some way he or she can get extra attention. Attention is an even more satisfying commodity to the young (or the middle-aged and old, for that matter) than ice cream, cake, and candy. Let your child pass out the forbidden food to others in much the same way that some alcoholics like to act as bartender at parties.

You can also give parties at your own home. That allows you to present approved food in such entertaining ways that neither your child nor the guests will realize, or care, that they aren't getting the junk food their hearts desire.

As for Halloween, your first decision is whether to allow your child out at all. If you do, and he or she comes home with a bag of loot, ADA board member Netti Richter, writing in *Diabetes Forecast*, offers some good suggestions:

> Why not help sort out the acceptable healthy foods and save a few sugary ones for handling reactions? What about the rest of the candy? In our house the garbage disposal is a great eater of "nondesirable foods."
>
> Knowing that resisting candy will be rewarded by an exchange gift at evening's end might make trick-or-treating less frustrating for a child. For example, exchanging the candy for a Halloween storybook at bedtime can be fun.

Use your own imagination to help your child stay on the diet instead of using your pity to allow him or her to break it "just this once."

Now, after having given the official party line, which happens to be our own opinion as well, here's a more lenient variation reported by a physician whom we respect, Dr. Lawrence

Power, author of the syndicated column "Food and Fitness" and consulting physician for National Health Systems (publishers of health reference charts).

A colleague of his who sees many diabetic children and young people says that a number of young diabetics, especially teenagers, who don't want to be different and who long for the fun foods their peers get to wolf down, totally rebel. They refuse to follow their diets and as a result stay constantly out of control.

This doctor makes a deal with the kids. If they promise to stick to their diet at all other times, they get six Hog Wild Days a year, six celebration days such as Christmas or their birthdays or graduation day, when, as far as food is concerned, anything goes.

"Do you know how high they usually kick up their heels on those days?" the doctor asks. "A Coke and a hamburger or a hot fudge sundae. Big deal."

Dr. Power himself adopted the Hog Wild Day method with his adult heart-attack patients. "Everyone needs a binge now and then," he says, "whether it's mint bonbons, Big Macs, or a cholesterol quiche. Something in most of us calls for a break from the routine. . . . There's room for the occasional departure for a holiday. It is the daily habits that get us into health mischief, not the occasional celebration."

Only you know your child well enough to decide whether the Hog Wild system would be a safety valve that would let off enough steam to allow him or her to simmer down to a good daily dietary routine or if it would only break down the already flimsy barriers against hazardous eating habits.

If you *do* opt for Hog Wildness, you should have a clear understanding with your child that the six days are to be spread out over the year and not clustered into an orgy week that could prove disastrous.

Should I send my child to diabetes summer camp?

Unless your child is the kind who would be miserably homesick and suffer psychological damage at *any* summer camp, we think it's a good idea—especially for younger and newly diagnosed children. We've had reports from young people who consider their camp experience a breakthrough in understanding their diabetes and in learning new practical techniques of management. Even more important to them was the realization that they're not oddballs and that the world is full of other diabetics who are successfully coping with the condition.

It's a genuine comfort for a diabetic to be in a situation in which virtually everyone is a diabetic and the nondiabetic is the one who's peculiar. Barbara had this latter experience one day at one of the SugarFree Centers. June and Ron, both diabetic, were on the scene, as was our cleaning woman, another diabetic. (We practice reverse discrimination and hire diabetics when we can.) Everyone who dropped by that day was diabetic. Even the mail was all from diabetics. Barbara began to get the creepy feeling that she was the only nondiabetic on earth and that there was something wrong with her for *not* having it.

Summer camp is also a good way for a child who has perhaps been overprotected at home because of diabetes to develop self-reliance.

One major benefit of diabetes summer camp is for the parents. For a short while you get out from under the stress and strain of worrying about your diabetic child. You know he or she is in the best of hands and you can get away for a little R and R yourself. You need it and you deserve it. Stress works its damage on you as well as on the diabetic child.

Summer camp can also give you a chance to improve your relationship with any nondiabetic in the family. They may be developing feelings of being less loved because they don't get the constant concern that the diabetic child gets. A week or two of exclusive attention can be a booster shot of security and self-esteem for them.

We have heard a few complaints about diabetes summer camps, including one from a mother whose already too-thin child came home five pounds lighter and showing ketones, and from a young woman who was disturbed and disgusted by the wild goings-on with alcohol and marijuana in one camp for teenagers. But these are isolated instances. The overwhelming majority of the reports have been favorable.

What can we do if we can't afford all the costs involved with our child's diabetes?

There is help available in the form of Supplemental Security Income (SSI). This is a federal program that makes monthly cash payments to disabled people who don't own much in the way of property or other assets and who don't have much income. Diabetes counts as a disability. A child's SSI payment can be as much as $477 a month, although some may get less because of their parents' income.

For further information, and for instructions on how to file, call the SSI office at 800-234-5772.

I just can't get my husband (wife, friend, etc.) to take care of his (her) diabetes no matter how hard I try. Is there anything I can do?

Unfortunately, you're not alone. Many people are desperate about trying to get those they love to take care of their diabetes and themselves. We frequently receive letters like the following, written by a young man:

> I have been involved with a wonderful lady name Sheila. About a year and a half ago we learned that she is a Type I diabetic. We are always considering marriage, but I must admit I'm frightened about our future together. Her problem is not the fact that she is diabetic. She has been fighting a losing battle with a severe sugar addiction. It has nearly destroyed our relationship many times, and she becomes so depressed that it is really unbearable. She desperately wants to beat this addiction to sweets, but nothing has seemed to work for more than a day or two at a time. There is

some progress, but I fear that time is quickly running out. Sheila has already noticed a decrease in her vision as well as constant poor circulation. Her diabetologist dropped her as a patient because she was not doing what he told her. It's evident that these sugar binges of hers could prove fatal.

I love Sheila with all my heart and soul and want so much to beat this damned disease and have as much of a future as God would permit us. Such a wonderful person as Sheila deserves as full a life as possible. I hope she can take control of this disease before it takes control of her.

We also get some success stories. For example, we received the following note, which came attached to an announcement of graduation from law school:

We got our meter from you in December. Since then my husband's diabetes has been controlled. It certainly took a load of worry off my mind during my last year in law school. In that light I wanted to share my graduation with you.

One young woman confessed to us that her husband told her that she used to be disagreeable about half the time, but since she started controlling her blood sugar, she's become "a wonderful human being and a joy to be around."

You might have your spouse or friend read the above so he or she could see what a shattering—or positive—effect a diabetic's control can have on loved ones. You could express your feelings. Even if he or she isn't willing to control the diabetes for himself or herself, he or she might start doing it to free you and the rest of the family from worry and allow you all to live your lives to the fullest.

But if spouses or friends should decide to control their blood sugar for the benefit of others, they should also investigate why they don't want to control it for themselves. Don't they consider themselves worth the effort? Don't they love themselves enough? If the answer is no, they may have a real problem, a problem more serious than diabetes and one for which they should seek professional counseling.

What is a remission?

A remission is a period when diabetes becomes less severe. For example, an insulin taker might find that he or she can stay in control on less insulin or on diet and pills, or maybe even on diet alone. Or perhaps a pill taker can get by on diet alone. Sometimes a remission lasts quite a while. Sometimes it is short-lived.

Particularly common is the "honeymoon period" remission that occurs in juvenile diabetes after insulin treatment begins. This often causes the parents, who are already desperately clutching at straws, to think their child has been miraculously cured or that the diagnosis of diabetes was incorrect. False hope. Diabetes is still there. A remission is *not* a cure and should never be regarded as such. Enjoy it while it lasts, but realize it will eventually end, and don't be devastated when it does.

My husband (wife, friend, etc.) wants to think and talk about diabetes all the time. What can I do?

It's hard to find a middle-of-the-road diabetic. Diabetics either try to ignore the disease totally or become almost obsessed by it. Those who fall into the obsessive category are at least better than the ignorers. They'lll probably live longer and eventually outgrow their obsession.

As a matter of fact, many diabetics are obsessed only for a while, right after they're diagnosed. It's not surprising that they should be preoccupied when they first confront a disease that demands the constant attention and thought that diabetes does. Much of the diabetic's talk about diabetes at this time is just musing out loud as he or she tries to figure out what to do;

whether he or she needs another slice of bread to make up for that yard work before dinner; if those funny feelings indicate low blood sugar or if they're something totally unrelated to diabetes.

One way that might tone a diabetic down a little is to become more informed about diabetes yourself. By showing the diabetic that you know something about diabetes, he or she may begin to feel less desperate about the subject and relax and let you do some of the thinking. If the two of you have workable, give-and-take exchanges on new solutions to diabetic problems, perhaps he or she will be able to cut the personal, lonely fretting time in half and start to think and talk about something else.

Your advantage in knowing something about diabetes is that when it is the subject of discussion, you'll understand what the person is saying. Then the talking will seem a lot less like a foreign language you don't understand, and, consequently, it will be a lot less boring to you.

If this plan doesn't work or just seems to feed the person's obsession, you may eventually have to get tough. Tell him or her in no uncertain terms that nobody loves a monomaniac and that the obsession only alienates people. This won't be easy to do, especially if you have sympathy and love for the diabetic. Unless somebody sets him or her straight, however, the person is going to ruin his life by thinking of himself as a walking case of diabetes rather than a human being with infinite interests and infinite possibilities who just happens to have diabetes.

How can I tell if a diabetic has low blood sugar?

It helps if you know the diabetic well enough to recognize behavior that isn't normal. If a generally easygoing person starts snapping and snarling, it may be low blood sugar. If a decisive person becomes vague, that can be a clue. Fumbling hands, glassy eyes, slurred speech, perspiration on the forehead or upper lip, a dopey smile, an odd, taut look about the face—all can be symptoms of hypoglycemia. Just about all diabetics have some signs peculiar to themselves that you'll grow to recognize if you're around them a lot and are observant.

Even if you know the person well, though, it's not always easy to recognize low blood sugar. We still remember the time we were talking to the Glendale chapter of the Diabetes Association of Southern California and told about one of our editors who said she could always recognize when June had low blood sugar "because she starts being mean to Barbara." We noticed a woman in the audience frowning. During the question-and-answer period she said, "My little boy has diabetes and takes insulin. Often, in fact, *very* often before dinner he's a holy terror. I can't do a thing with him. Could that be low blood sugar?"

"Oh boy, could it!" we chorused.

She was really shaken, because she had been punishing him for what was likely a misbehavior of his chemicals.

When you ascertain that a diabetic does have low blood sugar, take action immediately (see page 155). Above all, don't follow the example of the sister of a diabetic friend of ours, who, when she saw he was starting to act funny, looked terrified and announced, "You've got low blood sugar! I'm getting out of here!" And she fled.

How can I keep from getting mad at my roommate when he's obnoxious because his blood sugar is low?

It's tough not to get mad. You're human, too, and sometimes you have a visceral reaction that you can't control. Just do your best to keep calm enough to help your roommate get out of the reaction, even if he fights you on it.

After the incident is over you'll probably both laugh about it. Once June had low blood sugar and became furious because she thought Barbara had eaten her dish of strawberries (which she had actually eaten herself, but couldn't remember). After her

anger came despair, as she wept over her disappointment about
the strawberries she had so looked forward to. With a baleful
look at Barbara, she kept wailing, "You stole my strawberries."
Throughout all this wrath and woe, she steadfastly refused to eat
anything else to bring up her blood sugar because "the only thing
I wanted was those strawberries and you ate them." In retrospect,
the incident seems funny to us, but while it was going on it was
like a scene out of Eugene O'Neill. At such times you feel you're
dealing with an insane person. (Of course, you are.) So never
take seriously or bear a grudge over something a diabetic says or
does when in hypoglycemia.

You have one big advantage in this situation: You know
what low blood sugar is and can usually recognize it. This puts
you way ahead of the average person. Think how people who
know nothing about diabetes must react when confronted by your
roommate's obnoxious behavior.

I don't like to be impatient with all the things the diabetic has to do to take care of his or her diabetes, but I admit that sometimes I am. Is there anything I can do about it?

All of us with diabetic friends or family members want them to
take good care of themselves and stay healthy so we'll enjoy their
love and companionship for years. And we know that taking care
of diabetes takes time—lots of it. We know this intellectually but
not always emotionally. For example, sometimes we're ready to
go out to dinner or a movie or a sports event, and we have to stop
and wait for a blood-sugar test or a snack or some diabetic
something-or-other. We may get impatient, even irritated. We're
not upset with the diabetic person, of course. It's the diabetic
condition that bugs us. Still, the diabetic person is receiving a
negative message, even if it's being delivered in a silent language.

You don't like yourself for your impatience with diabetes routines, but you can't help it. Or can you? It's possible for you to turn these moments of time that diabetes steals from you into moments that you steal for yourself. All you have to do is figure out some things you really want to do, and reserve these stolen moments to do them. You can read a book. You can work a crossword puzzle. You can play a musical instrument. You can do needlework. You can meditate. You can practice magic tricks. You can do anything that doesn't take a lot of time to set up.

If you get in the habit of truly enjoying the diabetic-routine time, it will help both you and the diabetic be happy. You may even start hearing yourself say, "Are you sure you don't want to test your blood sugar before we go out?"

What am I likely to do that will irritate my diabetic companion most?

Remember the old Paul Simon song "Fifty Ways to Leave Your Lover"? Well, there must be 150 ways to irritate your diabetic. In fact, if that diabetic takes insulin and you catch your friend when he or she has low blood sugar, anything you do, including trying to get him or her to eat something to raise his or her blood sugar, can irritate or even enrage him or her. (Some diabetics in that state have even been known to hurl food into the face of the person trying to help.)

All diabetics, even when their blood sugar is normal and even if they don't take insulin, have their pet peeves. You'll just have to find out with experience what they are.

We can start you off with a few tips, though. A diabetic hates to hear the same phrase over and over from you. For example: "Is that on your diet?" "Did you remember to take your injection?" "Did you bring along a snack?" Anything you keep repeating begins to grate after a while.

June, for some reason, gets furious when asked, "Do you

have low blood sugar?" (She claims Barbara always asks this in an accusatory tone.) Her response is usually a garbled con-glomeration of "How should I know?" "Do you see a blood-sugar sensor sticking into me that I can read?" "Do you want me to stop what I'm doing and take my blood sugar; is *that* what you're saying?" Rant. Rant. Rant. She actually prefers to be told, "You're acting weird" or asked, "Why are you being so obnox-ious?" probably because it's not the oft-repeated phrase that she's come to loathe.

Nagging, which one psychologist defines as "trying to con-trol with criticism," is also near the top of the diabetic irritation scale. Nagging is not only irritating to a diabetic but also a futile endeavor on your part. Changes are going to be made only when the diabetic wants to make them. The best that you can do is to help him or her climb Maslow's hierarchy of needs (see Diabetes and Your Emotions: "How do I start making all the changes I have to for my diabetes?" on page 37) to the point that change is possible.

Another thing that will bother your diabetic friend is your cadging snacks. Insulin-taking diabetics need to carry sweets at all times in case of an insulin reaction. If friends who are aware of this storehouse of goodies persist, like Goldilocks, in eating them all up, the diabetic can be in trouble in an emergency.

A far, far better thing to do is to find out what your friend likes for diabetic snacks and carry something at all times for emergencies (and for your own snacking).

Probably the number-one irritant for diabetics is a lack of effort on your part to understand diabetes. Among her close friends June has some she's known for years and in whose homes she has frequent meals. All of them have supposedly read most of our books, and yet they still have only a vague idea of what she can and cannot eat. They understand little about how her meals must be scheduled or what to give her when she has low blood sugar. Since these friends are not stupid, she can only infer that they don't really care. A feeling that your friends don't care goes deeper than irritation. It goes into the hurtful-wound area.

If I mention my friend's diabetes in a restaurant to try to get her something special, like a substitute for sweet-and-sour pork in a Chinese dish, she gets furious and says I make her feel like a freak. What can I do?

The answer is simplicity itself. You say to the waiter, "I am a diabetic and I can't eat anything with sugar in it. Could we please substitute pork with Chinese greens for the sweet-and-sour pork?" By claiming to be the diabetic yourself, you take the burden of asking for special favors off your friend's conscience, or pride, or whatever area of his or her pyschological being is disturbed.

After you've claimed to be the diabetic for a while, maybe your friend will awaken to the fact that having diabetes is nothing to be ashamed of. He or she will come to realize that for the most part, people in restaurants as well as in other walks of life are usually happy to help out with little problems associated with diabetes. This is an important step in his or her acceptance of the disease.

What should I do if we're out dining in a restaurant and my friend, who is diabetic, orders all the wrong things?

Diabetics sometimes perversely do this. Even June, who is the most careful and rational of diabetics, has occasionally suffered this restaurant aberration.

The best thing to do when you hear the diabetically inappropriate meal being ordered is *not* to screech and rant and embarrass your friend in front of the waiter, but rather to order a diabetic backup meal for yourself. Usually when the diabetic's meal is presented to him or her, the diabetic takes one look at it and comes to his or her senses. Then you just say casually, without any lectures or recriminations, "It looks as if my dinner might be better for you than yours. Would you like to trade?" The diabetic almost always will with gratitude, probably as much gratitude for the freedom from lectures and recriminations as for the food.

Naturally, to perform this little sleight-of-plate act, you have to know what a diabetically appropriate meal is. So read the diet sections of this book on pages 42−52.

How do I plan a meal for my diabetic friend?

Just remember that a diabetic has to stay away from concentrated sweets—sugar, honey, and molasses in or on foods, and canned fruit in sweet syrup. Many diabetics also have to restrict the amount of fat they eat. Remember also that diabetics, especially those who take insulin, need a specific amount of carbohydrate in their diet. Just have something like bread, rice, pasta, or potatoes available, and the diabetic will know how much of it to eat.

That's another point to remember. Just as important as what is allowed is how much. A diabetic must eat limited quantities of food. Don't be offended if your diabetic friend eats with gusto and then suddenly stops, as if someone has blown a whistle. There isn't a bug in the food or anything. It's just that the diabetic has eaten all that's allowed. Don't urge him or her to have more. That's being cruel. The diabetic would probably love to eat more, and it's taking every ounce of willpower to stop.

A basic diabetic meal would be something like this: a mixed green salad; chicken or fish or meat; potatoes or bread or pasta or rice; a vegetable or two; and fruit for dessert (either fresh or canned without sugar). Now, on the surface this may sound pretty bland, but any and all of these elements can be combined in something like beef stroganoff or bouillabaisse or chicken marengo or lamb curry. Just remember, generally, what ingredients you put into the dish and tell the diabetic so he or she can estimate portions. As for drinks, read the information on alcohol (see page 72). If you're still confused about anything on the diabetic diet, just follow the advice of all the sex-manual writers who say, "If in doubt about what will please your partner, *ask!*"

If your diabetic friend is on insulin (ask!), you should indicate at what time you're serving. This doesn't mean what time the guests are arriving but what time you'll actually have everybody sitting at the table with food on their plates. Then, once you've set the time, *stick to that time,* no matter who hasn't arrived by then (unless, of course, it's the diabetic who's late).

Should I give up eating pastries so my diabetic roommate won't feel tempted?

Admittedly, it's a little hard to sit there and wolf down a huge slab of banana cream pie if your roommate is watching you like a spaniel. You both feel sorry for him or her, you feel guilty, and these are very digestion-upsetting emotions. Still, you definitely shouldn't give up your pastries for your roommate's sake. He or she is going to have to get used to being tempted and resisting temptation. It's similar to an alcoholic's situation: he or she has to be able to go to a place where others are drinking and yet not drink.

There remains, however, a question you didn't ask. And that is, Should you give up pastries for your own sake? Pastries are hardly the nutritional dream dish for anybody, diabetic or not. And how is *your* weight?

My son wants to play football. Is that safe for a diabetic?

There have been several outstanding diabetic football players. Ron Mix of the University of Southern California and Coley

O'Brien of Notre Dame are just two. Many high-school football players shared their experiences with us when we were writing our previous books. No diabetic evil ever befell them because of football. If your son's diabetes is without complications and under good control and his doctor doesn't disapprove, then there is no reason he shouldn't play.

There are two good reasons he should. Participation in sports, especially a physically demanding one like football, will encourage him to take superb care of himself and his disease. For a young person, the incentive to keep in shape for football is far more powerful than a general incentive to watch one's health. Once your son has established good habits during his football-playing days, there's a fair chance he'll stick with them throughout his life.

He should be allowed to play football for psychological reasons as well. If his diabetes keeps him from playing football, he'll get the idea that because of diabetes he can't do anything.

On the other hand, if he plays football, his attitude will more likely be that, despite his diabetes, he can do everything he really wants to. Which attitude would you prefer him to carry through life?

Be sure he informs the coach and his teammates that he has diabetes and explains to them what they should do in case he has an insulin reaction.

And finally, do your best not to show excessive concern every time he goes out to play, even if you feel it way down inside your own pancreas. If you load him up with fears and negative feelings, you'll wreck his game and maybe cause an accident rather than prevent one. A football players needs a positive attitude above all else, and so does a diabetic.

Note: One case in which we feel you're justified in forbidding your son to play football is if your family doesn't believe in the violence of the sport and none of your children is allowed to play it. In that case it would be wrong to bend over backward and let your diabetic son do something you don't let the others do.

Should I give my brother his insulin injections?

Yes and no. Yes, you should give them to him sometimes. You can reach injection sites he can't reach himself, unless he's a contortionist. This is a big help.

Another reason for giving him his insulin is that you'll know how to give an injection. Should he ever pass out in insulin shock, you'll know how to give him glucagon (see page 202), which is injected in the same way as insulin, and bring him out of it.

But no, you shouldn't *always* give him his injection. He's got to be mainly responsible for his own insulin shooting. No one should be that dependent on another person. It's almost like being dependent on another person for your breathing. It's not good for him or for you, either.

What's the best way to celebrate a diabetic's birthday or other special occasion?

It takes some ingenuity and foresight to create the kind of birthday celebration that's best for a diabetic. Fortunately, there are now sugar-free baking and frosting mixes available. If you keep those on hand, you'll always be ready to make something for birthday parties and other special occasions. Check with the local bakeries. As part of the diabeticization of America that we've been talking about, many bakeries are adding sugar-free cakes to their repertoires. (We know of four in the Los Angeles area.) You can even be truly original and make something like a sandwich cake. It looks like a cake, but when you cut into it, it's actually a club sandwich frosted with something like blended cottage cheese and yogurt.

When it comes to gifts for diabetics, you should heed the excellent advice given in the journal *Diabetes Self-Management*, by Charles Mallory, a Kansas City free-lance writer who has a diabetic wife:

Don't make every gift related to diabetes. Treats don't always have to be sugar-free candy or dietetic chocolates, nor does a Christmas gift have to be a health-club membership or dinner out at the new low-calorie restaurant. Your wife probably likes flowers, traveling, clothes, and entertaining. Your husband may like cufflinks, cologne, or a greeting card for a special occasion. None of these has to do with diabetes. Wouldn't you be disappointed if, at a birthday party, your friends who knew you were Catholic gave you nothing but Virgin Mary statuettes and rosary beads?

What should I do if I were to find a diabetic unconscious?

Unconsciousness can be due to either diabetic coma, which means the diabetic has extremely high blood sugar, or insulin shock, which means it's extremely low. If you know the diabetic takes insulin and sticks to his or her diet pretty well, then you can be almost certain it's insulin shock.

First, never under any circumstances pour any liquid like fruit juice or Coca-Cola down an unconscious diabetic's throat, as it could wind up in his or her lungs and cause suffocation. The only thing you can do, if you've had good instruction and know where it is, is give an injection of glucagon. Otherwise, call the paramedics or a doctor. A word to the thrifty: an injection of glucagon costs about $25; calling the paramedics can cost over $400.

If you know for sure that the diabetic doesn't take insulin and/or doesn't follow the diet or take care of him or herself, then it's probably a diabetic coma, the result of long-range diabetic misbehavior. In this case, call the doctor or an ambulance immediately. There's nothing much you can do in this kind of crisis. Only a hospital can help now.

If you have no idea whether you're dealing with insulin shock or diabetic coma, treat for insulin shock. If it's diabetic coma, the diabetic already has so much sugar floating through his or her system that a little more isn't going to make all that much difference. And if it *is* insulin shock, your quick treatment could be a lifesaver. A person in good health will eventually come out of insulin shock spontaneously, but for someone with a heart condition the shock could be life threatening.

Reference Section

. . . .

Medications that increase blood-glucose levels

Chlorthalidone
Corticosteroids
Diazoxide
Furosemide
Epinephrinelike medications
Estrogens
Nicotinic acid
Phenytoin
Syrups containing sugar
Thyroid preparations
Thiazide
Glucagon
Caffeine (large quantities)
Cyclophosphamide
Ethacrynic acid
Asparaginase
Morphine
Nicotine
Lithium

Medications that lower blood-glucose levels

Ethyl alcohol
Insulin
Sulfonylureas
Beta blockers
Anabolic steroids
Fenfluramine
Biguanides
Salicylates (large doses)
Disopyramide
Phenobarbital (and other
    enzyme inducers)

Directory of Organizations

American Association of Diabetes Educators
500 N. Michigan Ave., Ste. 1400
Chicago, IL 60601
312-661-1700
Write for information on diabetes education programs and a list
of certified diabetes educators in your area.

American Diabetes Association
1660 Duke St.
Alexandria, VA 22314
800-ADA-DISC
Write for the address of your local chapter if it is not listed in
your phone book.

American Dietetic Association
216 W. Jackson Blvd., Ste. 800
Chicago, IL 60606-6995
312-899-0040
Can provide names of qualified dietitians in your area.

Juvenile Diabetes Foundation International
432 Park Avenue South
New York, NY 10016-8103
800-223-1138
A national group whose objective is to fund research aimed at
curing diabetes and preventing its complications. Information,
educational programs, and meetings for diabetic children and
young people and their families. Write for address of your local
chapter.

SugarFree Centers for Diabetics
13715 Burbank Blvd.
P.O. Box 114
Van Nuys, CA 91408
Centers in various locations; mail-order service. Diabetes self-

care equipment and products, books, educational materials, and gourmet health foods. Call for location of centers and for free newsletter. Nationwide except California 800-972-2323; California: 800-336-1222.

How Sweet It Is

Aspartame	A protein sweetener 180 times as sweet as sucrose. Technically, aspartame is caloric; however, it is so sweet that the amount used per serving of food is likely to supply almost no calories. Marketed as Equal and NutraSweet.
Carob Powder Carob flour	Produced by grinding the pod of the carob tree. Tastes similar to chocolate. Seventy-five percent is made up of sucrose, glucose, and fructose, which are all caloric.
*Cyclamates**	*Noncaloric* sweeteners approximately thirty times as sweet as sucrose. Cyclamates were banned from use in the United States in 1970 because of questions about their possible cancer- and tumor-causing properties. They are still used in some foreign countries, and the risk associated with moderate use is considered by many to be very small. In 1989 it was announced that the U.S. ban on cyclamates was being lifted and that cyclamates would again be available.
Dextrin	Chains of glucose molecules. Their effect on blood glucose has not been well evaluated but may be similar to glucose. Caloric.
Dulcitol	A sugar alcohol. Caloric.
Fructose Fruit sugar Levulose	One of the most common naturally occurring sugars, particularly found in fruit and honey. It is not associated with a rapid and high rise in blood sugar in well-controlled diabetes. The sweetness of refined fructose varies, but under certain conditions it can be almost twice as sweet as sucrose. Caloric.

*The sweeteners in italics are generally felt to be appropriate sweeteners for the diabetic individual, provided they are used according to the recommendation of a physician or dietitian.

Glucose
  Corn sugar
  Dextrose
  Grape sugar
	A naturally occurring sugar that normally causes a fast and high rise in blood sugar. About half as sweet as table sugar. Carbohydrates (starches) break down to glucose during digestion, as do all sugars eventually. Glucose is the form of sugar that the body uses for energy and other purposes, and it builds up in the blood if diabetes is poorly controlled. *Dextrose* is the commercial name for glucose and will often be seen on food labels, including those of some sugar substitutes. Caloric.

Glucose Syrups
  Corn syrup
  Corn-syrup solids
  Sorghum syrup
  Starch syrup
  Sugar-cane syrup
	Liquid sweeteners produced by the breakdown (hydrolyzation) of starch. They contain a mixture of glucose, maltose, and longer chains of glucose molecules and can be produced from a variety of starches (hence, the varied names). *Corn-syrup solids* are the crystallized form of corn syrup. Caloric.

High-Fructose Corn Syrups	Produced from corn syrups. They contain differing amounts of fructose, ranging from 42 to 90 percent. The remaining part of the syrup is primarily glucose. The effect of the highly refined type (90 percent fructose) on blood glucose has not been well evaluated, but, theoretically, it should not cause high and fast rises of glucose in the blood of people whose diabetes is well controlled. The 90 percent type is the only one that might prove to be an acceptable sweetener for diabetics. Caloric.

Honey
  Comb honey
  Creamed honey
	A natural syrup that varies in sugar and flavor depending on many factors. It is primarily glucose (about 35 percent), fructose (about 40 percent), and water and, by weight, is about 75 percent as sweet as sucrose. Additional glucose is sometimes added to some honeys. Caloric.

Lactose	Milk sugar. It comprises about 4.5 percent of cow milk. About 30 percent as sweet as sucrose. Caloric.

Maltose	Two glucose units linked together. It is only 30 to 50 percent as sweet as sucrose, but it rapidly breaks down to glucose in the intestinal tract. Caloric.
Mannitol	A naturally occurring sugar alcohol that causes less of a rise in blood sugar than do sucrose or glucose. It is about half as sweet as sucrose and is slowly absorbed into the blood. In large amounts, it can cause diarrhea. Caloric.
Maple Syrup Maple sugar	Made from the sap of the maple and other trees. It is mostly sucrose, with some invert sugar (see *sucrose*) and trace amounts of other compounds. The crystallized syrup is *maple sugar*. Caloric.
Milk Chocolate Bitter chocolate Bittersweet chocolate	Produced by the addition of milk, sugar, and cocoa butter to bitter chocolate. *Milk chocolate* is approximately 43 percent sugar and *bittersweet chocolate* is about 40 percent sugar. The sugar is caloric.
Molasses Blackstrap Golden syrup Refiners' syrup Treacle Unsulphured	The sugar drawn from sugar crystals as they are refined into pure sucrose. Different types are usually produced during sucrose refinement. All types, however, contain 50 to 75 percent sugar (sucrose and invert sugar) and should generally be avoided by diabetics. The sugars are caloric.
Saccharin	The currently used *noncaloric* sweetener in the United States. It is about 375 times as sweet as sucrose.
Sorbitol	A naturally occurring sugar alcohol found in many plants; commercially produced from glucose. It is about half as sweet and more slowly absorbed than glucose. In individuals whose diabetes is well controlled, it causes only a small postmeal rise in blood glucose. In large amounts it may cause diarrhea. It is widely used in the manufacture of dietetic foods and chewing gums. Caloric.

Sucrose
  Beet sugar
  Brown sugar
  Cane sugar
  Confectioner's
    sugar
  Invert sugar
  Powdered sugar
  Raw sugar
  Saccharose
  Sugar
  Table sugar
  Turbinado
	A naturally occurring sugar that is composed of equal parts of glucose and fructose linked together. It is produced from sugar cane or sugar beets. *Invert sugar* is made of sucrose that has been broken down to equal parts of glucose and fructose (with some sucrose left intact). *Brown sugars, raw sugar,* and *Turbinado* all contain some molasses.

Sweetened
  Condensed
    Whole Milk
  Sweetened
    condensed
    skim milk
  Sweetened
    condensed
    whey
	Produced by reducing the water content of milk by about half and adding sugar. The finished product is about 44 percent sucrose, which is caloric. This means a fourteen-ounce can of condensed whole milk contains the equivalent of eight tablespoons of sugar and two and a half cups of milk.

Xylitol	A naturally occurring sugar alcohol produced from xylose (bark sugar). It is slowly absorbed and causes less of a rise in blood sugar than does sucrose or glucose. Depending on how it is used, it is as sweet as or less sweet than sucrose. It is believed to be less cavity inducing than other sugars. Large amounts can cause diarrhea, and questions about its safety have held up its use in all but a few products. Caloric.

Carbohydrate and Caloric Values of Alcoholic Beverages

Beverage	Amount	Calories	Grams of Carbo-hydrate
Ale, Beer			
Ale, domestic	8 ounces	104	8
Beer, domestic	8 ounces	114	10³/₅
Champale	8 ounces	127	10
Cocktails, Premixed			
Black Velvet (Heublein)	1 ounce	65	0
Daiquiri (Calvert)	1 ounce	63	3
Daiquiri (Heublein)	1 ounce	59	4
Daiquiri (Hiram Walker)	1 ounce	59	4
Manhattan (Calvert)	1 ounce	54	³/₄
Manhattan (Hiram Walker)	1 ounce	49	1
Margarita (Calvert)	1 ounce	59	3
Margarita (Heublein)	1 ounce	48	2
Martini (Calvert)	1 ounce	59	0
Martini (Heublein)	1 ounce	56	²/₅
Martini (Hiram Walker)	1 ounce	56	¹/₄
Old-Fashioned (Hiram Walker)	1 ounce	55	1
Vodka martini (Hiram Walker)	1 ounce	49	0
Whiskey sour (Calvert)	1 ounce	65	3
Whiskey sour (Hiram Walker)	1 ounce	59	4
Distilled Spirits*			
80 proof	1 ounce	67	0
84 proof	1 ounce	70	0

*Bourbon, brandy, cognac, Canadian whiskey, gin, rye, rum, scotch, tequila, vodka.

Beverage	Amount	Calories	Grams of Carbo-hydrate
Distilled Spirits (*cont.*)			
86 proof	1 ounce	72	0
90 proof	1 ounce	75	0
94 proof	1 ounce	78	0
94.6 proof	1 ounce	79	0
97 proof	1 ounce	81	0
100 proof	1 ounce	83	0
Liqueurs, Cordials			
Akvavit (Aalborg Regular)	1 ounce	62	⅛
Akvavit (Aalborg Jubilaeums)	1 ounce	62	2½
Anisette (Bols)	1 ounce	111	14
Anisette (Hiram Walker)	1 ounce	92	10¾
Apricot cordial (Hiram Walker)	1 ounce	82	8⅕
Apricot-flavored brandy (Hiram Walker)	1 ounce	88	7½
Blackberry brandy (Bols)	1 ounce	100	7⅖
Blackberry cordial (Hiram Walker)	1 ounce	100	12¾
Blackberry-flavored brandy (Hiram Walker)	1 ounce	86	7
Blackberry liqueur (Bols)	1 ounce	96	9
Cherry cordial (Hiram Walker)	1 ounce	82	8
Cherry Heering (Hiram Walker)	1 ounce	80	10
Crème de cacao (Bols)	1 ounce	101	11⅘

Beverage	Amount	Calories	Grams of Carbohydrate
Liqueurs, Cordials (*cont.*)			
Crème de cacao (Hiram Walker regular or white)	1 ounce	104	15
Crème de menthe (Bols)	1 ounce	112	13
Crème de menthe (Hiram Walker green or white)	1 ounce	94	11⅕
Crème de noyaux (Bols)	1 ounce	115	13¾
Curaçao (Bols blue)	1 ounce	105	10⅓
Curaçao (Bols orange)	1 ounce	100	8⅘
Curaçao (Hiram Walker orange)	1 ounce	96	11¾
Drambuie (Hiram Walker)	1 ounce	110	11
Ginger-flavored brandy (Hiram Walker)	1 ounce	72	3½
Irish Mist	1 ounce	120	5⅗
Kümmel (Hiram Walker)	1 ounce	71	3¾
Peach cordial (Hiram Walker)	1 ounce	81	8
Peach-flavored brandy (Hiram Walker)	1 ounce	87	7⅕
Peppermint schnapps (Hiram Walker)	1 ounce	78	7⅕
Rock and rye (Hiram Walker)	1 ounce	87	9½
Sloe gin (Bols)	1 ounce	85	4¾
Sloe gin (Hiram Walker)	1 ounce	68	4¾

Beverage	Amount	Calories	Grams of Carbo-hydrate
Liqueurs, Cordials (*cont.*)			
Southern Comfort	1 ounce	120	3½
Tia Maria (Hiram Walker)	1 ounce	92	10
Triple sec (Bols)	1 ounce	113	8⅘
Triple sec (Hiram Walker)	1 ounce	105	9¾
Wines			
Champagne, brut	3 ounces	75	1
Champagne, extra dry	3 ounces	87	3¾
Dubonnet (Schenley)	3 ounces	96	7
Marsala (Florio dry)	3 ounces	162	18
Marsala (Florio sweet)	3 ounces	182	23
Mirin (Kiku-Masamure)	3 ounces	225	36
Port, Ruby	3 ounces	138	10
Port, Tawny	3 ounces	138	11
Red table wine (dry)	3 ounces	69	trace
Sake (Kiku-Masamure)	3 ounces	75	6
Sherry, dry	3 ounces	120	1
Sherry, sweet	3 ounces	150	6
Vermouth, dry	3½ ounces	105	1
Vermouth, sweet	3½ ounces	167	12
White table wine (dry)	3 ounces	74	trace
Mixers, Soft Drinks			
Bitter lemon (Schweppes)	10 ounces	160	39⅖
Bitter orange (Schwepps)	10 ounces	153	37¾
Catawba sparkling grape juice	3 ounces	58	14¾

Beverage	Amount	Calories	Grams of Carbo-hydrate
Mixers, Soft Drinks (*cont.*)			
Club soda (Schweppes)	10 ounces	0	0
Ginger ale (Schweppes)	10 ounces	110	27
Ginger beer (Schweppes)	10 ounces	120	29²/₅
Lime juice (Rose's sweetened)	1 ounce	49	12
Moxie	10 ounces	129	29
Tonic water (Schweppes)	10 ounces	110	27½

Courtesy of Ida Jaqua, Professor Emeritus, Los Angeles Valley College.

Target Heart Rates

Age	20	25	30	35	40	45	50	55	60	65	70
Maximum Heart Rate	200	195	190	185	180	175	170	165	160	155	150
85% of Maximum Heart Rate	170	166	162	157	153	149	145	140	136	132	128
80% of Maximum Heart Rate	160	156	152	148	144	140	136	132	128	124	120
70% of Maximum Heart Rate	140	137	133	130	126	123	119	116	112	109	105

Doctor's Initial Examination

On your first visit to a new doctor or shortly thereafter, you should undergo a comprehensive evaluation of your diabetes. The following components are an indispensable part of that evaluation.

Complete History and Physical Examination

Although the history is probably the most important feature of the initial evaluation, full details cannot be provided here for space reasons. Essential points that should be covered include family history of diabetes; circumstances at the onset of the diabetes; history of treatment through diet, exercise, pills, and insulin; and evaluation of the effectiveness of current treatment. In addition, the presence of or potential for diabetic complications should also be reviewed. These complications are macrovascular (arteriosclerosis affecting circulation to the heart, legs, and brain); microvascular (affecting the retina and kidney); and neuropathic (leading to numbness in the feet, impotence, or other symptoms).

The physical exam should be as comprehensive as any you've ever had. Important aspects of the exam include:

■ *Blood pressure*. A risk factor for diabetic complications and a reflection of subtle changes in kidney function.

■ *Eyes*. Retinal exam to check for diabetic retinopathy.

■ *Neck*. Evaluation for autoimmune thyroid disease.

■ *Heart*. Check for macrovascular complications (arteriosclerosis) affecting circulation to the heart.

■ *Pulse*. Evaluation for arteriosclerosis. Pulse should be checked in the neck, wrists, groin, top of foot, and inner ankle.

■ *Neurological*. Check for sensations in the feet. "Reflexes" checked with a hammer tap at the ankle and knee.

■ *Feet.* Examination for pulse and neurological function as well as deformities such as bunions or hammer toes, calluses, breaks in the skin, and improperly cut toenails.

Laboratory Evaluation

The following tests are especially important in evaluating a patient with diabetes:

■ *Blood sugar.* A seemingly indispensible part of diabetes care, but is *one* blood sugar value really that important, compared with what the patient can test at home?

■ *Glycosylated hemoglobin.* Essential in evaluating overall diabetes control and as a baseline for further improvements in therapy.

■ *Cholesterol, HDL Cholesterol, triglycerides.* Total cholestrol and LDL Cholesterol (calculated from the three lipid tests) are used to evaluate the risk of diabetic macrovascular complications. Triglyceride values (which are often elevated in diabetes) may also reflect the level of overall diabetes control.

■ *Creatinine.* A measure of kidney function, not especially sensitive to early changes. Measuring "creatinine clearance" by obtaining both a blood test and a twenty-four-hour urine specimen is much more sensitive.

■ *Urinalysis.* Important as a screen for infection and to look for urine protein.

■ *Microalbuminuria.* The most sensitive measure for early diabetes kidney effect, this test should become the standard for patients with diabetes. It can be measured with a random, overnight, or twenty-four-hour urine collection.

■ *Urine culture.* Should be done if the urinalysis shows any abnormality.

■ *Thyroid function tests.* Essential for every patient with Type I diabetes to be screened for autoimmune thyroid disease.

■ *Electrocardiogram (EKG).* Should be done routinely in patients who are over forty or who have had at least ten years of diabetes. A baseline reading is often done on all patients at the first visit.

These data form the basis of your initial evaluation and, in a shortened version, may become the model for a yearly diabetes update. But remember—medical care cannot be evaluated by a checklist; your own physician may have a different way of organizing the above data. Still, one way or another, this information should be part of every diabetic patient's record. Knowing what to expect, and what data to ask for, will help you become more informed about your own health and medical care.

Recommended Reading

· ·

Basic Books on Diabetes

Bernstein, Richard K., M.D. *Diabetes: The GlucograF™ Method for Normalizing Blood Sugar*. Los Angeles: Jeremy P. Tarcher, 1981. Dr. Bernstein, a Type I diabetic for forty-two years, is known as "the tartar of tight control." His scientific method requires six self-tests a day, multiple injections of insulin, and a high-protein diet. This pioneer book is of great value to Type I diabetics who are tired of their bouncing blood sugars and are ready to take charge of their diabetes to prevent complications and to feel their best twenty-four hours a day.

Biermann, June, and Barbara Toohey. *The Diabetic's Total Health Book*. Los Angeles: Jeremy P. Tarcher, 1988. First published in 1980, this book proves that you can have a chronic disease and yet be a picture of health, leading a vital, productive, and happy life. It shows you how to do it by focusing on your health rather than on your disease. It teaches you how to achieve a strong body, a tranquil mind, and a blithe spirit. The new edition is thoroughly up-to-date to reflect the latest changes in diabetes therapy and diet.

Diabetes A to Z. Alexandria, Va.: American Diabetes Association, 1989. An outstanding mini-encyclopedia that covers almost everything everyone ought to know about lifestyle, nutrition, exercise, and any other subject you might need to have more information about. Written in easy-to-understand terms, with complete discussions of every subject covered.

Jovanovic, Lois, M.D., June Biermann, and Barbara Toohey. *The Diabetic Woman.* Los Angeles: Jeremy P. Tarcher, 1987. The first book to focus on how women can best deal with diabetes at different stages of their lives, both therapeutically and emotionally. Women have always felt more alone with diabetes than men, because of the distinctive complexity of their diabetes-related problems. There is support and understanding here as well as realistic coping methods for the major and minor concerns in the lives of today's women. Special chapter for family members.

Krall, Leo, M.D., and Richard Besser, M.D. *Joslin Diabetes Manual.* Philadelphia: Lea and Febiger, 1989. The new twelfth edition of the manual from Boston's famed Joslin Clinic. A kind of postgraduate course for diabetics who want to know all the hows of diabetes care and the scientific whys behind them. Wonderfully up-to-date coverage, clearly presented, with many handy charts and tables. Perfect as a home reference guide.

Lodewick, Peter, M.D. *A Diabetic Doctor Looks at Diabetes.* Waltham, Mass.: RMI Corporation, 1988. In this complete manual Dr. Lodewick is always optimistic and understanding and never preachy. He gives you the very latest in diabetes therapy—his own therapy. He shares with you the experiences of some of the thousands of diabetic patients in his practice. Newly revised.

Lowe, Ernest, and Gary Arsham, M.D. *Diabetes: A Guide to Living Well.* Diabetes Center, Inc., 1989. This book helps you design a program of individualized self-care on whichever level you are comfortable with: intensive, moderate, or loose. Chapters on stress, diet, emotions, and exercise. Special sections for women and children. One author has had diabetes for thirty-five years and the other for forty years. A very distinctive and informative book.

Mirsky, Stanley, M.D., and Joan Heilman. *Diabetes: Controlling It the Easy Way*. New York: Random House, 1982. In this book Dr. Mirsky, a highly experienced endocrinologist of Mount Sinai School of Medicine in New York, shares his expertise and positive views.

Monk, Arlene, et al. *Managing Type II Diabetes*. Minneapolis: International Diabetes Center, 1988. A simple how-to guide for people who have non-insulin-dependent diabetes. Written by a team of experts, this easy-to-read manual provides a thorough explanation of, and the most current information about, this type of diabetes.

Moore, Michael, ed. *Learning to Live Well with Diabetes*. Minneapolis: International Diabetes Center, 1985. A comprehensive, easy-to-understand manual on all aspects of diabetes care. Thirty chapters written by twenty-four prominent medical and health-care experts.

Peterson, Charles, M.D., and Lois Jovanovic, M.D. *Diabetes Self-Care Method*. New York: Simon and Schuster, 1984. A state-of-the-art manual that focuses on normalizing blood sugar through self-testing and insulin adjustment. The physicians who wrote this book believe most complications can be avoided; included is a chart telling which are preventable and which are reversible. A very practical and encouraging book by two of the foremost endocrinologists in the United States.

Sims, Dorothea F., ed. *Diabetes: Reach for Health and Freedom*. St. Louis: C. V. Mosby, 1984. Sims is a leader in diabetes education and is herself an inspiring role model with forty-one years' experience as a diabetic. She edited this self-care manual written by a team of health professionals. It emphasizes options rather than rules. A large portion of the book is devoted exclusively to the problems of Type II diabetics. Compassionate and supportive.

Cholesterol Control

Cooper, Kenneth, M.D. *Controlling Cholesterol.* New York: Bantam Books, 1988. This is an authoritative postgraduate course in cholesterol and triglyceride control. Dr. Cooper cites an impressive number of scientific studies to confirm his beliefs. As you would expect from a fitness expert like Dr. Cooper, the exercise section is particularly outstanding. Includes menu plans and recipes with exchanges.

Kowalski, Robert E. *Eight-Week Cholesterol Cure.* San Francisco: Harper and Row, 1987. Start with this book if your cholesterol is over 200. It presents a proven program for lowering your cholesterol by up to 40 percent by using oat bran and niacin (a B vitamin). Oat bran also has excellent weight-reducing and blood-sugar-lowering capabilities for diabetics. (Check with your doctor about niacin.) Fast improvement guaranteed, yet the plan is not a dogmatic joy killer. Use sugar substitutes for the sugar, honey, etc. in the recipes. Excellent chart of calories, fat, cholesterol, and sodium in brand-name and fast foods.

Kraus, Barbara. *Cholesterol Counter.* New York: Putnam, 1985. An index to thousands of brand-name and basic foods, giving their cholesterol count by portion size. Includes foods that do not contain cholesterol as well as those that do.

Cookbooks and Exchange Lists

ADA Family Cookbooks. 3 vols. New York: Prentice-Hall, 1980, 1984, 1987. These three cookbooks are healthy eating guides for the entire family, not just for diabetics. Volume 1 has 250 recipes, information on nutrition, meal planning, exchanges, dining out, and fast food. Volume 2 has 206 recipes, four chapters on fighting fat, an exercise program, ethnic dishes and exchanges, plus a section on fiber. Volume 3 focuses on variety and popular dishes such as tortilla soup, fajitas, and jambalya. Features quick-cooking tips; microwaving method included when appropriate. All recipes are reduced in fat, are low in sodium, and are limited to a half-teaspoon sugar.

Anderson, James, M.D. *Diabetes: A Practical New Guide to Healthy Living; HCF Guide Book; HCF Exchanges.* New York: Warner Books, 1981. Lexington: HCF Diabetes Foundation, 1978, 1988. These three books explain Dr. Anderson's High Carbohydrate Fiber (HCF) nutrition plan, which he began studying and developing in 1974. The plan is particularly helpful for overweight non-insulin-dependent diabetics. The HCF diet can lower insulin requirements and eliminate the need for pills in many Type II diabetics. The HCF diet has lately come into prominence because it also lowers cholesterol. In fact, Dr. Anderson is the original oat-bran enthusiast. *Diabetes: A Practical New Guide to Healthy Living* deals with the treatment of diabetes. The *HCF Guide Book* gives directions for using the diet plan and contains many tips for microwaving, shopping, eating out, etc. It also contains recipes and sample menus. The *HCF Exchanges* is an expanded list of the eight exchange groups used in the plan.

Bailey, Covert. *Fit or Fat Target Diet; Fit or Fat Target Recipes.* Boston: Houghton Mifflin, 1984, 1985. These are the follow-up books to Bailey's fitness and weight-loss plan explained in *Fit or Fat?* The first is an eating plan emphasizing losing body fat. The second is a collection of recipes for delicious, low-fat dishes ideal for weight control for Type II diabetics.

Barrett, Andrea. *The Diabetic's Brand-Name Food Exchange Handbook,* rev. ed. Philadelphia: Running Press, 1989. Calories and exchanges for three thousand foods from four hundred manufacturers plus ten fast-food menus. Vital for those with fast-lane eating habits.

Exchange Lists for Meal Planning. American Diabetes Association and American Dietetic Association, 1986. Food lists created by the American Diabetes and Dietetic associations to help diabetics control calories and eat balanced diets. A dietitian can tailor the lists to your needs.

Exchange Lists for Weight Management. American Diabetes Association and American Dietetic Association, 1989. Exchange lists especially for those who need to lose weight.

Finsand, Mary Jane. *The Diabetic Candy, Cookie, and Dessert Cookbook.* New York: Sterling Publishing Company, 1982. Chemist-nutritionist Finsand gives you over two hundred recipes using sugar replacements. A treasure of thrills for dessertees. Even tells you how to make ice-cream cones. Contains twelve pie recipes, seventeen cake recipes, and forty-four cookie recipes. Don't overdo! (But then don't underdo, either!)

————. *The Diabetic Chocolate Cookbook.* New York: Sterling Publishing Company, 1984. The luxury of chocolate in candies, cookies, cakes, pies, and puddings is here made possible for diabetics. Exchanges and calories are provided for each recipe.

————. *The Diabetic High-Fiber Cookbook.* New York: Sterling Publishing Company, 1985. A first! High-fiber cookery just for diabetics and their families. Covers the entire menu. Lots of vegetable recipes, soups, stews, and casseroles. An entire chapter on making sausages from different countries, many with bran flakes or cornmeal. Contains two hundred and fifty recipes, all with calorie counts and exchanges.

Franz, Marion. *Exchanges for All Occasions.* Waysata, Minn.: Diabetes Center, Inc., 1987. Revised in 1987, this manual lists hundreds of foods not on the ADA exchange lists. Covers high-fiber, vegetarian, and ethnic diets. Essential for flexibility in dining.

Gilliard, Judy, and J. Kirkpatrick. *Guiltless Gourmet.* Waysata, Minn.: Diabetes Center, Inc., 1987. By a dietitian and a diabetic trained in classic French cuisine. This book has sophisticated recipes from all over the world, all computer analyzed for the diabetic diet. All are low in fat, cholesterol, sugar, and calories.

Healthy Food Choices. American Diabetes Association and American Dietetic Association, 1986. An introductory eleven-by-seventeen-inch poster to help you get started on an ideal meal plan by making the right food choices in the right amounts. Folds into a booklet.

Jacobson, Helen. *Special Diet Foreign Phrase Book.* Emmaus, Pa.: Rodale Press, 1982. Use this book to explain what you want in Spanish, French, German, or Italian. It covers all diets—diabetic, low sodium, low cholesterol and fat, ulcer, bland, soft and low residue. The print is large enough so that you can point to the phrase and let the waiter or maître d' read it. Includes medical-emergency phrases and everything else you need to make your trip healthful and fun.

Jones, Jeanne. *The Calculating Cook: More Calculated Cooking.* San Francisco: 101 Productions, 1972, 1981. Written by a famous cook and diabetic who specializes in good food that's good for you. This book makes dining a joy. All recipes include exchanges.

Kahn, Ad. *Diabetes Control and the Kosher Diet.* Skokie, Ill.: Wordscope Associates, 1984. The only book about managing diabetes in accordance with Orthodox Jewish religious practices. Besides three chapters of recipes there are lower-fat and calorie adaptations of traditional dishes such as chopped liver and matzo balls. Includes Kosher exchange lists.

Kruppa, Carole. *Free and Equal Sweet Tooth Cookbook.* Chicago: Surrey Books, 1988. One hundred and fifty new quick and delicious low-calorie desserts and sweet treats, all using the sweetener Equal (NutraSweet). These recipes are also low in salt and cholesterol. Exchanges and calories are given.

Little, Billie, and Victor Ettinger, M.D. *Gourmet Recipes for Diabetics.* New York: Putnam, 1987. Just what the title says. Contains one hundred and forty-seven recipes for the adventurous by an expert cook and an epicurian endocrinologist. Their motto: Stay on the Diet, but Enjoy! Enjoy!

Majors, Judith S. *Sugar Free Good and Easy; Sugar Free Goodies; Sugar Free Kids' Cookery; Sugar Free Microwavery.* Milwaukie, Ore.: Apple Press, 1985, 1987, 1987, 1980. Finally back in print, four books approved by the Oregon affiliate of the ADA and written by a diabetic woman who confesses she "lives to eat." All recipes are simple and quick. *Goodies* is for those with a sweet tooth—pies, cookies, jams, ice creams (1986 ADA exchanges). *Good and Easy* has breads, salads, main dishes—everything for variety and good meals (1976 exchanges). *Kid's Cookery* has recipes with child appeal that are simple enough for young diabetics to prepare (1986 exchanges).

Marks, Betty, and Lucille Schechter. *International Menu Diabetic Cookbook.* New York: Contemporary Books, 1985. Betty Marks (a diabetic) and Lucille Schechter make foreign cooking possible for diabetics. They present an amazing variety of exotic but easily prepared dishes that are not high in fat. Contains three hundred recipes from eighteen countries, along with seventy-three menu suggestions. Includes exchanges, sources of foreign ingredients, and helpful hints.

Methven, Barbara. *Microwaving Light and Healthy; Microwaving on a Diet.* Minnetonka: Cy DeCosse, 1985, 1981. A microwave oven is a dieter's—and a diabetic's—best friend, making cooking fast and easy. Both books have mouth-watering illustrations and lip-smacking recipes, and both explain menu planning and include recipes from appetizers to desserts, with calories, sodium, cholesterol, and exchanges.

Middleton, Katharine, and Mary Hess. *Art of Cooking for the Diabetic.* New York: Contemporary Books, 1988. An excellent choice for your first diabetes cookbook. This total food guide is by a diabetic diet counselor and a nutrition educator with diabetes in the family. Completely updated with the latest nutritional advice. Contains three hundred and fifty recipes that are low in sugar, saturated fat, and sodium.

Pennington, Jean, and Helen Church. *Food Values of Portions Commonly Used.* San Francisco: Harper and Row, 1989. The fifteenth edition of the bible of nutrition. Gives complete nutrient content of all foods—and we do mean all. Essential for dietitians and people on special diets.

Reader, Diane, and Marion Franz. *Pass the Pepper, Please!* Waysata, Minn.: Diabetes Center, Inc., 1988. Hypertension is twice as common in diabetics, so they especially need to reduce sodium. This book tells how to eliminate salt without tears and almost without effort.

Revell, Dorothy. *Oriental Cooking for the Diabetic.* Tokyo: Japan Publications, 1981. At last a dietitian has opened up Oriental cooking to diabetics. Includes all the old favorites of Chinese and Japanese cuisine—egg-flower and miso soups, egg foo yong, tempura, sweet-and-sour pork, etc. Many recipes use the stir-fry method. The exchange values of all special Oriental ingredients are given—even quail eggs and whale meat. There is a group of recipes for those who are on a sodium-restricted diet. Includes calories and exchanges for each dish.

Robertson, Laurel, Carol Flinders, and Brian Ruppenthal. *The New Laurel's Kitchen.* Berkeley: Ten Speed Press, 1986. *Laurel's Kitchen* has always been our favorite vegetarian cookbook. The new *Laurel* has the same inspiring philosophy and new recipes that open vistas of dining joy and health. Tells how to increase fiber and cut back on fat. Sections on cooking for children, elders, pregnant women, and athletes.

Wedman, Betty. *ADA Holiday Cookbook.* New York: Prentice-Hall, 1986. A collection of marvelous low-sugar, low-salt, low-fat recipes for traditional holiday favorites like roast turkey, eggnog, fruitcake, pumpkin treats, challah, and gefilte fish. Also many

appealing dishes that you can enjoy all year long, like pumpkin
pancakes, popovers, etc. Includes tempting vegetarian creations.
Exchanges given from the 1986 ADA lists.

Emotional Health and Stress

Edelwich, Jerry, and Archie Brodsky. *Diabetes: Caring for Your
Emotions.* New York: Addison-Wesley, 1986. This book explores
the deepest feelings of diabetics. It is told in the words of the
people who lived through them. Outstanding chapters on sex-
uality, conflicts with health professionals, and family dynamics.
Type II diabetics, who often get short shift, are given as much
attention as Type I's.

Burns, David, M.D. *Feeling Good.* New York: New American
Library, 1980. Psychiatrist David Burns shows how by changing
the way you think you can alter your moods and get rid of low
self-esteem, anger, depression, pessimism, lethargy, and the other
"black holes" in your life and become rich in self-assurance,
strength, and accomplishment.

Biermann, June, and Barbara Toohey. *The Peripatetic Diabetic.*
Los Angeles: Jeremy P. Tarcher, 1984. Our first and most personal diabetes book, the one that tells how to overcome that
initial fear and despair and move on to a more joyful, exciting,
and healthy life than ever before. This edition was recently updated with a section called "The Peripatetic II," to bring you into
the contemporary world of diabetes therapy. But the original
book with all of its crises and confusions is still there, exactly as
it was written—and lived.

Parents and Children

Ducat, Lee, and Sherry Suib Cohen. *Diabetes Guide for Parents.*
San Francisco: Harper and Row, 1983. The full subtitle of this
book is *A New and Complete Guide to Healthier Living for*

Parents, Children and Young Adults Who Have Insulin-Dependent Diabetes. This is a real coping manual, and it is outstanding on the emotional aspects of diabetes. Lee Ducat has a diabetic son and is the founder of the Juvenile Diabetes Foundation International.

Loring, Gloria. *Kids, Food, and Diabetes.* New York: Contemporary Books, 1986. Because of her diabetic son, TV star Gloria Loring was inspired to write an exceptional book that only a sensitive, caring mother could. It's packed with recipes that kids will love, sound nutritional information, and, best of all, lots of Loring's personal suggestions for coping with the challenges of raising a diabetic child while keeping the dynamics of good family relationships intact. Like having your own support group right on your bookshelf.

Roberts, Willo Davis. *Sugar Isn't Everything.* New York: Macmillan, 1987. The subtitle of this novel is *A Support Book, in Fiction Form, for the Young Diabetic.* A professional children's book writer who herself became diabetic as an adult, Willo Roberts turned her own new knowledge and experience into a factually sound, therapeutically up-to-date novel with an eleven-year-old girl as its heroine. Amy develops diabetes, struggles with it, learns how to handle it, and eventually accepts it. Engrossing and true to life. Every young diabetic can relate to this novel, and learn more and feel better for having read it. Good for parents, too.

Siminerios, Linda, and Jean Betschart. *Children with Diabetes.* American Diabetes Association, 1986. By two experienced and dedicated diabetes nurse-educators of the Children's Hospital of Pittsburgh. This manual for parents is concise yet complete, covering treatment (insulin, diet, exercise, testing), emergencies (hypoglycemia, hyperglycemia, diabetes coma, sick days), and problems special to babies, preschoolers, school-aged children, and adolescents. Gives parents insights into emotional problems and suggestions for the entire family.

Magazines

Countdown, 432 Park Avenue South, New York, NY 10016-8013; 800-223-1138. The magazine of the Juvenile Diabetes Foundation International. Published four times a year. Subscription price $16.

Diabetes, 1660 Duke St., Alexandria, VA 22314; 800-232-3472. Published by the American Diabetes Association, this is a journal for members of its professional section. Published monthly. Subscription price $50.

Diabetes Care, American Diabetes Association, 1660 Duke Street, Alexandria, VA 22314; 800-232-3472. A scientific research journal that publishes articles on research in the field of diabetes. Subscription price $55.

The Diabetes Educator, 500 N. Michigan Ave., Ste. 1400, Chicago, IL 60611; 312-661-1700. The journal of the American Association of Diabetes Educators. Published bimonthly. Subscription price $35.

Diabetes Forecast, American Diabetes Association, 1660 Duke St., Alexandria, VA 22314; 800-232-3472. Magazine for diabetics. Published monthly. Subscription price $18 (included in your membership dues of $24, if you join the ADA).

Diabetes in the News, Ames Center for Diabetes Education, Miles, Inc., Diagnostics Division, 224 E. Monroe, South Bend, IN 46601; 312-664-9782. Magazine for diabetics. Published bimonthly. Subscription price $9. (Address subscriptions to P.O. Box 3105, Elkhart, IN 46515.)

Diabetes Self-Management, R. A. Rapaport Publishing, Inc., 150 West 22nd St., New York, NY 10011; 201-391-6306. Magazine for diabetics. Published bimonthly. Subscription price $18. (Address subscriptions to P.O. Box 51152, Boulder, CO 80321-1125.)

Index